APPALACHIAN
MENTAL HEALTH

APPALACHIAN MENTAL HEALTH

Edited by

SUSAN EMLEY KEEFE

THE UNIVERSITY PRESS OF KENTUCKY

Editorial and Sales Offices: Lexington, Kentucky 40506-0336

Library of Congress Cataloging-in-Publication Data

Appalachian mental health / edited by Susan Emley Keefe.
   p. cm.
   Includes bibliographies and index.
   ISBN 0-8131-1614-7 (alk. paper)
   1. Rural poor—Mental health—Appalachian Region, Southern.
2. Rural poor—Mental health services—Appalachian Region, Southern.
3. Rural poor—Appalachian Region, Southern. 4. Appalachian Region,
Southern—Rural Conditions. I. Keefe, Susan E. (Susan Emley)
   [DNLM: 1. Mental Health. 2. Mental Health Services—Appalachian
Region. 3. Social Environment—Appalachian Region. WM 30 A646]
RC451.4.R87A67 1988
362.2'042'0974—dc 19
DNLM/DLC
for Library of Congress   88-20557

Contents

IV. CULTURAL CONSIDERATIONS IN
THERAPEUTIC ENCOUNTERS

V. PROBLEMS AND PROMISE IN APPALACHIAN
MENTAL HEALTH SERVICE DELIVERY

Tables

Figures

Preface

This book is intended as a guidepost in an as yet ill-defined field. Pioneering works in Appalachian mental health were introduced in 1971 by David H. Looff and Robert Coles, but it is difficult to identify a larger body of literature on the topic. This collection of articles makes the literature more accessible as it reviews many of the findings of researchers from a variety of disciplines. The collection also presents new data gathered by researchers including anthropologists, sociologists, psychologists, psychiatrists, and social workers, using methodologies ranging from interviews to surveys to clinical data collection forms. These data and the experience of the authors, who have done research or provided therapeutic services in the region, form the basis for a multitude of recommendations for the improvement of mental health services in the mountains. These are summarized in the introductory and concluding chapters. If this collection also serves as an impetus for further research and the practical application of findings on mental health in Appalachia, it will have achieved yet another intended goal.

This book grew out of a symposium on mental health in Appalachia organized by Warren Johnson at the annual meeting of the Summer Study Program on Rural Mental Health Services, in Madison, Wisconsin, in 1981, and a follow-up workshop, organized by Keefe in 1982, on Appalachian mental health at Appalachian State University, which was attended by practitioners from around the region. Preliminary versions of the chapters by Beaver, Cole, Efird, Humphrey, and Keefe were presented at one or both of these conferences. At these and subsequent workshops and programs relating to mental health in Appalachia, it has become apparent that there is a growing interest in a regional perspective on mental health and culturally relevant techniques that can be incorporated easily into clinical practice. This collection has been directed to both academically inclined researchers and practicing professionals in the region. It is hoped this alliance will continue and lead to further developments in the field of Appalachian mental health.

A collection of this sort is always a group effort. I would like especially to thank Patricia Beaver who, then director of the Center for Appalachian Studies at Appalachian State University, first invited me to participate in a discussion of mental health in Appalachia at an in-service training program in 1980 and who helped in organizing the workshop held at ASU in 1982. I would also like to thank the Department of Anthropology and the College of Arts and Sciences at Appalachian State University for giving me time to devote to this project. Teresa Isaacs has patiently and attentively typed the manuscript; her help is always greatly appreciated. Finally, I am lucky to have a supportive and loving family and I must thank my husband, Tom, and Megan and Rosemary, who have helped in so many ways as I have worked on this book.

Introduction

SUSAN EMLEY KEEFE

This collection of articles addresses mental health issues in Southern Appalachia. There are two very good reasons for such a book. In the first place, the Appalachian region suffers from significant problems and deficiencies in the delivery of mental health services. Appalachia is underserved by mental health professionals and services, as are most rural areas in the United States (see Efird, Chapter 9); but because Appalachia covers one of the largest and poorest rural populations in the country, its need is intensified. Moreover, the mental health facilities that do serve the region tend to be located in urban centers, creating problems in accessibility for rural and low-income residents. Social, economic, and cultural factors—including high rates of poverty and unemployment, low levels of education, widespread occupational and environmental hazards, and the lack of complete integration into the national social and cultural fabric—would seem to indicate the potential for higher rates of stress and a greater need for mental health services. Yet, there is apparent underutilization of the services that exist.

In the second place, there is general agreement that Appalachians as a people are different and therefore deserve special consideration as distinct from mainstream Americans. The basis for this differentness is controversial. Some of the authors in this collection see mountaineers as a separate ethnic group. Others concentrate on the largely rural and/or lower- and working-class nature of the region's population. Certainly, Appalachians share many traits with the rural poor as well as with ethnic minority groups elsewhere in the nation. Like these groups, the people of Appalachia have experienced historical patterns of control and exploitation (reviewed by Beaver, Chapter 1). In fact, several authors compare the relationship of Appalachians and mental health services to other systems of control in the region (see Van Schaik, Chapter 6; White, Chapter 14; and Sovine, Chapter 15). If nothing else, then, Appalachia as a region is clearly the product of a unique historical experience of inequality, and its people have been set apart in both symbolic and material ways from the rest of America.

The "differentness" of Appalachia has often been conceptualized as cultural and reputed implications about the significance of cultural difference have been at the heart of the debate concerning the relationship between Appalachia and the rest of America. Therefore, this essay first addresses the interpretation of cultural difference used by earlier writers in the field of Appalachian mental health and the current need for critical studies using a more informed concept of culture. Second, it summarizes the content of the articles in this collection, focusing on the distinctiveness of the Appalachian experience as it comes to bear on mental health issues. The implications for regional mental health services and future research are discussed in the concluding chapter of the book.

THE NEED FOR CRITICAL STUDIES

Appalachia has not been dealt with in a tolerant or even-handed way by either the larger society or academic scholars. The past century of exploitation of the region's rich natural resources has been accompanied by a wholesale condemnation of the people and their culture. This has occurred not only in the popular media, beginning with the local color writers of the late nineteenth century (see Shapiro 1978), but also in the academic literature, where Appalachians have been described variously as "barbarians" (Toynbee 1947), "yesterday's people" (Weller 1965), "regressive" (Polansky, Borgman, and De Saix 1972), and "nonrational" (Ball 1968). The correlation of political, economic, and cultural domination of the area has been well documented cross-culturally, and work in the last decade, especially by Gaventa (1980) and Whisnant (1983), serves to demonstrate the nature of this relationship between the dominant society and the regional periphery of Appalachia. The emergence of a critical literature concerning Appalachia and the perception of its people is the result, I believe, of real political and economic changes and a growing sense of power in the region. Symbolic of these changes, in a way, has been the emergence of scholars who are natives of the region and who have led in founding the new field of Appalachian studies. Furthermore, the research of recent years has done much to redress the negative portrayal of Appalachians and the inadequacy of previous analytical models used to interpret the region.

The field of Appalachian mental health, however, has yet to receive significant attention in the way of critical studies. This is surprising since the image of Appalachia presented by mental health studies prior to the mid 1970s is one of the most derogatory on record.

For the purposes of illustration, it is worth reciting some of these pejorative remarks that ultimately characterize the Appalachian people and their culture as deviant. As a consequence, the social, psychological, and economic problems evident in the region are blamed to a greater or lesser degree on this perceived cultural deviance. David Looff (1971), a child psychiatrist, is perhaps the most restrained of the authors to be discussed in his tendency to characterize Appalachian culture negatively. He recognizes the need to understand local culture from the participant's perspective and frequently demonstrates sensitivity and insight in portraying Appalachian people. Yet, in the end, he resorts to a culture-of-poverty interpretation of causation[1] and blames the "overly close families" of Appalachia for the various mental problems he sees in his eastern Kentucky clinic, including especially school phobias, overly dependent personality disorders, and conversion reactions. Looff attempts some balance in his approach, however, by noting, for example, the absence of certain disorders based to some extent on extreme emotional deprivation in infancy.

In the collection edited by psychologist and psychiatrist Joseph Finney (1969), we find a much greater tendency to type the entire "subculture" in the region as deviant; Finney himself, in the introduction, labels Appalachia a "culture of conversion reaction or hysteria." One of the participants at the conference on which the volume (Finney 1969) is based, Rena Gazaway, presents a description of a "sick" community in eastern Kentucky characterized by chronic poverty and hopelessness (see also Gazaway 1969), a community that fellow conference participant Oscar Lewis accepts as having a "culture of poverty." In an instructive discussion following Gazaway's presentation, disagreement emerges among the participants regarding the idea that the people of "the Branch" are mentally ill and the relative significance of internal versus external causes of their maladjustment. The study by social workers Polansky, Borgman, and De Saix (1972), on the other hand, contains no such qualifications. The authors summarily list a number of cultural themes in Appalachia that are judged in a clinical sense to be "regressive," including dependency, delusions of fusion (that is, unity), inexpressiveness, and fatalism. These perceived cultural predispositions lead to the development of an "apathy-futility syndrome," which Polansky et al. find characterizes the low-income mothers they studied in western North Carolina and north Georgia.

Two of the most derogatory and stereotyped pronouncements about Appalachian people are found in articles by sociologist Richard Ball (1968) and psychiatrist Charles Goshen (1970). Ball labels southern Appalachia "an analgesic subculture" distinguished by nonrational "frustration behavior" that is not goal oriented and includes traits marked by fixation, regression, aggression, and resignation. Ball relies on rat studies in experimental psychology and an environmental model to support his claims. Goshen, in contrast, offers no outside sources to support his description of two lower classes he identifies in Appalachia. He characterizes the lowest class of "cultural primitives" or "hillbillies" as "fundamentally uncivilized people" with "infantile speech," "weird, primitive" religion, frequent drunkenness and violence, and "clannish" families whose boundaries are blurred by illegitimacy and incest. The second lowest class of "traditional farmers" Goshen judges to be of better peasant stock but still pathologically unambitious. His diagnosis that these two classes of people are in a psychiatric sense "schizophrenic" and "psychoneurotic," respectively, would be laughable if it were not for the fact that the article appears in a medical journal.

All of these studies, which include some of the major works on Appalachian mental health, share a similar approach in that they blame the Appalachian people, their life-style, and their values for the poverty and mental illness found in the region rather than recognizing the institutions and processes deriving from the larger society that significantly shape conditions found in Appalachia. In addition, these studies tend to couch their cultural bias in psychiatric and clinical language, characterizing Appalachian people and culture in general with terms such as *conversion reaction syndrome* or *apathy-futility syndrome*, and as being *delusional*, *schizophrenic*, or *neurotic*. Not only are these presumptuous judgments based on limited studies, usually of the most isolated and poverty-stricken people and communities in the region, but because they employ medical terminology and are often written by authors having medical training, the studies take on the cloak of "science" and may be accepted uncritically as objective and factual.

In the collection of essays in this volume, a perspective on mental health in Appalachia is provided that portrays the people and culture of the region in a much more positive and balanced way than has been done in the past. Moreover, the authors in general recognize the broader social, political, and economic context in which Appalachian mental health must be evaluated. Finally, the volume provides a cumulative critique of the culture-of-poverty approach as it has shaped mental health studies in Appalachia.

PROFITING FROM THE CONCEPT OF CULTURE

One of the unfortunate consequences of the attack on the culture-of-poverty model in Appalachian studies has been to reject the concept of "culture" in favor of political and economic factors stemming from the larger society, which broadly define the way of life in Appalachia. Yet, it is imperative to recognize the importance an informed concept of culture can bring to understanding and improving the region's human services, including mental health care. *Culture*, in the anthropological sense, refers to a set of ideas and behavior that is learned, patterned, and transmitted from generation to generation. No culture is unique; each shares some traits with other cultures at a similar level of social organization. Moreover, cultural groups that share geographic boundaries, historical experiences, or ethnic heritage often are alike in many ways. Nevertheless, the pattern of traits that characterizes a particular cultural group emerges as distinctive and enduring.

Thus, life in rural Appalachia, marked as it is by egalitarianism and a concern for "neighborliness" and reciprocal exchange, has much in common with life in other rural areas of the United States, especially the rural South, and, indeed, with small-scale farming societies everywhere. Similarly, poverty and economic disadvantages have the same effect on Appalachians as they do on other peoples, causing, for example, feelings of powerlessness and a concern for present time as opposed to planning for the future. The qualities, however, that distinguish Appalachia as a cultural region stem more from the relatively homogeneous national origin of settlers in the eighteenth and nineteenth centuries, the majority being immigrants from Great Britain, and from a common historical experience, especially the extractive nature of early industrialization and the relative social isolation until the mid-twentieth century. Cultural traits such as a regional dialect (Wolfram and Christian 1976), a common religious orientation (Ford 1962), and the significance of the large "family group" in regional kinship organization (Brown 1952) help to create the distinctive nature of Appalachia. Moreover, the opposition perceived by and between Appalachians and "outsiders," fueled by positive feelings of cultural pride as well as pejorative stereotypes, contributes to differences in identity.

Where the culture-of-poverty model goes wrong, then, is in designating traits of socioeconomic origin as valued cultural patterns and, furthermore, attributing final causation to the culture. An understanding of cultural differences leads to a better understanding of the context within which groups of people interact and adaptively change through time. In terms of mental health, it can reveal the client population's perception of how and why people get sick and methods of appropriate treatment, all of which can differ from the mental health professionals' understanding of the process. "Culture" necessarily remains a mediating factor in explanatory models, however; it is not usefully conceptualized as the final cause of behavior.

Culture-of-poverty writers have not been alone in their tendency to designate Appalachian culture as "final cause" in trying to interpret the behavior of people in the region. Health and mental health professionals in Appalachia may also resort to blaming the culture for any difficulty in administering treatment (see Sovine, Chapter 15). Alternatively, health practitioners may adopt and manipulate native cultural perceptions rather than recognize the social and economic origins of illness (see Van Schaik, Chapter 6). Either approach tends to obscure the nature of illness for both patient and health practitioner and can be used to justify a lack of professional action. A more informed concept of culture, on the other hand, can sensitize the therapist to the context of the patient's illness, improve patient-practitioner communication, and should empower both the patient and the mental health professional. What if, for example, Sovine (Chapter 15) asks, therapists in eastern Kentucky "began to relate their own employment insecurity to that of the Appalachian miners?"

APPALACHIANS AND MENTAL HEALTH

The authors of the articles in this volume find many ways to characterize Appalachians (in particular the rural lower class) that have relevance for mental health services. The traits can be grouped as characteristics of (1) the Appalachian sociocultural system in general and (2) the relationship between mountaineers and mental health services.

Aspects of the Appalachian sociocultural system that emerge as significant include mountain people's perceptions of institutions established and staffed by professionals from outside the region, the value system of mountaineers, their family organization and indigenous support systems, and their beliefs concerning mental illness and appropriate treatments.

According to several of the authors, Appalachians are more likely to perceive institutions, social agencies, and professional helping agents with fear and suspicion (Cole, Chapter 12; Humphrey, Chapter 3; Keefe, Chapter 8). Because of the historical inequalities in the nature of their interaction with outsiders and authorities, Appalachians have learned to approach with caution those who say they have come to help, including doctors, social workers, and therapists. Given that these professionals frequently are not native Appalachians, they bear the burden of being perceived by the local population not only as outsiders but also as different by culture and socioeconomic status. Class and cultural differences can create barriers to the perception of individual strengths, such as the positive self-images Fiene (Chapter 5) finds among the low-income women she interviewed. In addition, institutions and agencies are not only perceived as cold and bureaucratic, but they often are staffed and/or administered by outsiders who are culturally insensitive to the people and the region (see Plaut, Chapter 11). It is little wonder then that agencies, including mental health services, tend to be avoided by native Appalachians.

Many authors in this collection emphasize core values in Appalachia that affect social interaction and perceptions of the helping professions. Three interrelated values stand out: egalitarianism, individualism, and personalism. These stem in large part from Appalachians' rural "frontier" heritage and the distinctive religious system that developed in the mountains (see Beaver, Chapter 1; Humphrey, Chapter 3). Given an egalitarian ethic, there is a dislike of authorities and institutions that set out to control the rights and behavior of others. Although a social status hierarchy is evident even in the rural areas, the ideal of equality is the one expressed publicly. Those who set themselves apart as being higher in status are perceived as "uppity" and sanctions are imposed upon them. Individuals are admired and judged on the basis of their personal achievements and qualities. Self-reliant behavior is idealized; help is unacceptable if it appears to be "charity." In social systems where individuals loom large, social standing is implicitly tied to a face-to-face society. Individuals expect to be personally recognized and dislike impersonal treatment. In such a social system, "strangers" can have little impact.

Familism is also an important value among mountain people, and extensive kin networks are the basis for local social organization (see Keefe, Chapter 3). Kinship and religion tend to be strongly interwoven as extended families often attend the same church, and the small churches in rural areas are frequently linked to just one or two local kin groups. As Humphrey (Chapter 3) points out, family and religion provide the individual's identity and security in the mountains. They are also the basis for the informal helping system available to individuals who experience emotional problems. Individuals can also seek solace and healing through prayer and may turn to faith healing in times of crisis. Family members are always at hand for advice and support. Migration can disrupt family networks, creating stress, and attempts to maintain reciprocity despite geographic obstacles can create more stress (see Halperin and Slomowitz, Chapter 13). As Halperin and Slomowitz find, urban Appalachian migrants who deviate from the cultural pattern of moving to cities where they have kin may be more at risk for acquiring emotional problems.

Illness is an unwelcome visitor for all people, but it is perhaps more feared by rural laborers and the poor who are without health benefits and who depend heavily upon the fulfillment of daily physical tasks by household members. While all illness is feared, many of the following authors find that Appalachians perceive *mental* illness far more negatively. As a result, few native Appalachians acquire problems perceived as mental or emotional, instead experiencing their mental problems as physical problems and preferring medicine as treatment for the somatic symptoms (see Van Schaik, Chapter 6; White, Chapter 14). The adopted medical model leads to the expectation for an immediate diagnosis and "cure" with associated disappointment in failure to find quick relief (see Efird, Chapter 9; Humphrey, Chapter 3; White, Chapter 14).

Authors in this volume argue that there is differential use of mental health services by mountain people. Not only is there apparent underutilization, but certain segments of the population are more at risk in Appalachia. Keefe (Chapter 10) finds, for example, that men and the middle aged are more likely to use mental health services in Appalachia than in the mainstream American population. It is tempting to tie this to the recent processes of culture change in the mountains, in which rural men have suffered a loss in status by taking up low-paying "public work" while women have gained in status with the control of resources through wage-paying jobs. Keefe also suggests that as more and more non-Appalachians move into the region, mountaineers may find it more difficult to compete for access to mental health services when they are deemed necessary.

The indigenous help-seeking process in Appalachia also has an impact on mental health service utilization. As several of the authors point out, Appalachians are more likely to seek *informal* help for emotional troubles and to avoid institutions and agencies (Cole, Chapter 12; Efird, Chapter 9; Keefe, Chapter 8). This preference is tied to the strong local family networks and a value of "helping their own." Even in extreme cases of mental deficiency or handicap, institutional aid is often refused (see Humphrey, Chapter 3). It is quite likely that the stereotype of higher rates of mental retardation often associated with Appalachia is instead the result of a difference in approach to treatment, rural Appalachians preferring home care in the community (resulting in greater visibility) as opposed to care in a distant institution, which would mean virtual loss of contact with the family member. In the formal system of mental health referral agents and services, it is not surprising given the emphasis on somatic symptoms of emotional problems to find that physicians are significant interceptors and play a sensitive role in the help-seeking process (see Keefe, Chapter 8).

The culture-bound perception of the etiology of mental illness and appropriate treatment also affect mental health service utilization. Several authors point out that Appalachians are more likely to designate spiritual causes for emotional problems and therefore may be more likely to see the need for religion-based healing (see Humphrey, Chapter 3; Keefe, Chapter 8; Sovine, Chapter 15). Like cultural groups elsewhere, Appalachians experience certain illnesses that are not easily equated with prevailing psychiatric categories. Van Schaik (Chapter 6) explores the illness called *nerves*, which is not unique to Appalachia but, being associated with poverty and high-stress conditions, is common in the region especially among women. Again, physicians are key in the diagnosis and treatment of this culture-bound illness in Appalachia.

Finally, the authors in the following pages find that the encounter between therapist and client in Appalachian mental health clinics is affected by cultural differences. Therapists are often non-Appalachians with little experience in Appalachian culture. While, as Sovine (Chapter 15) points out, the cultural differences are often recognized, their existence may simply be used as an excuse for the failure of treatment rather than as the basis for creating effective treatment. As a result of cultural disparities, Appalachians may be diagnosed in ways different from mainstream Americans; Keefe (Chapter 10) suggests they are more frequently diagnosed as having severe problems. This may also have to do with a cultural sensitivity to certain kinds of symptoms. For example, Plaut (Chapter 11) suggests Appalachians may be more likely than non-Appalachians to experience visual hallucinations. In addition, authors find a preference among Appalachians for a particular kind of interaction style with therapists that is more egalitarian and personal in nature, reflecting core values in the region (see Humphrey, Chapter 3; Plaut, Chapter 11). Finally, Sovine (Chapter 15) reminds us that, in general, therapists in Appalachia as elsewhere have entered the profession genuinely concerned about caring for the mentally ill but that the structure of Community Mental Health Systems incorporates other demands such that therapists frequently find it impossible to be "both efficiently bureaucratic and effectively therapeutic."

The field of Appalachian mental health has gone largely unexplored and much of the literature available is marked by an explicit culture-of-poverty orientation. Taking various approaches, the contributors to this volume successfully overturn many assumptions held by previous writers concerning the mental health of people in Appalachia. And, whereas the heterogeneity of the region is acknowledged in the diversity of subareas and populations discussed, dominant themes emerge concerning Appalachia as a whole, as we are presented with a cumulative portrait of a strong regional culture with native support systems based on family, community, and religion. Therapeutic approaches that consider the implications of this cultural context are also examined. Moreover, inquiry is directed to the potential for conflict between Appalachian client and non-Appalachian practitioner and between regional culture and mainstream mental health services. Although it is impossible to cover all relevant subjects, the authors present a host of practical suggestions on ways to improve mental health care in the region. In fact, the primary strength of the collection lies in this combination of concern for theoretical and applied issues.

The following chapters have been organized into five parts. Part I provides background on Appalachian culture and general implications for mental health systems. Part II examines the relationship between specific social and cultural attributes (particularly gender, socioeconomic status and family ties) and mental health problems. In Part III, there is an investigation of the factors affecting the use of mental health services in Appalachia and ways to improve the planning of services. Part IV is concerned with the impact of cultural factors on the relationship between therapist and client in the Appalachian setting, in particular when it involves the non-Appalachian therapist and the Appalachian client. Part V focuses on institutions in the mental health system, how they are maintained and their effect on clients. As the papers in this final section demonstrate, change in mental health services in the Appalachian region will ultimately require policy decisions at administrative (perhaps regional and even federal) levels.

NOTES

1. Briefly, the culture-of-poverty model proposes that a certain proportion of the chronically poor develop a culture characterized by authoritarianism, fatalism, present-time orientation, suspicion of authority, a tolerance of pathology, feelings of helplessness and inferiority, etc. (O. Lewis 1959). According to this model, the cultural value and belief system that thus develops in poverty also contributes to its persistence. This model has been criticized at length in the general social science literature (e.g., Leacock 1970) as well as in Appalachian studies (e.g., H. Lewis 1970).

REFERENCES

Ball, R.A. 1968. A poverty case: The analgesic subculture of the southern Appalachians. *American Sociological Review* 33:885-95.

Brown, J.S. 1952. The conjugal family and the extended family group. *American Sociological Review* 17:297-309.

Finney, J.C., ed. 1969. *Culture change, mental health, and poverty.* Lexington: University of Kentucky Press.

Ford, T.R. 1962. The passing of provincialism. In *The southern Appalachian region: A survey,* ed. T.R. Ford, 9-34. Lexington: University of Kentucky Press.

Gaventa, J. 1980. *Power and powerlessness: Quiescence and rebellion in an Appalachian valley.* Champaign: University of Illinois Press.

Gazaway, R. 1969. *The longest mile.* New York: Doubleday and Co.

Goshen, C.F. 1970. Characterological deterrents to economic progress in people of Appalachia. *Southern Medical Journal* 63:1053-61.

Leacock, E.B., ed. 1970. *The culture of poverty: A critique.* New York: Simon and Schuster.

Lewis, H. 1970. Fatalism or the coal industry? Contrasting views of Appalachian problems. *Mountain Life and Work* 46(11):4-15.

Lewis, O. 1959. *Five families: Mexican case studies in the culture of poverty.* New York: Basic Books.

Looff, D.H. 1971. *Appalachia's children: The challenge of mental health.* Lexington: University Press of Kentucky.

Polansky, N.A., R.D. Borgman and C. De Saix. 1972. *Roots of futility.* San Francisco: Jossey-Bass.

Shapiro, H. 1978. *Appalachia on our mind: The southern mountains and mountaineers in the American consciousness,* 1870-1920. Chapel Hill: University of North Carolina Press.

Toynbee, A. 1947. *A study of history. II.* New York: Oxford University Press.

Weller, J.E. 1965. *Yesterday's people: Life in contemporary Appalachia*. Lexington: University of Kentucky Press.

Whisnant, D.E. 1983. *All that is native and fine: The politics of culture in an American region*. Chapel Hill: University of North Carolina Press.

Wolfram, W., and D. Christian. 1976. *Appalachian speech*. Arlington, Va.: Center for Applied Linguistics.

PART I

The Appalachian Context

1

Appalachian Cultural Systems, Past and Present

PATRICIA D. BEAVER

Appalachia is a distinct region of the United States, set apart not only by geography but also by history. An understanding of the historical experience is essential for any interpretation of modern-day problems and prospects in the region. This essay presents a brief historical overview of Appalachia and considers the implications for mental health services.

HISTORICAL PATTERNS OF DEVELOPMENT

Settlement of the southern Appalachian region was well under way by the late eighteenth contury. Progressive waves of Scotch-Irish and German settlers, coming first down the great valley of Virginian into the piedmont areas of the eastern states, and later through southern ports, were joined by families of English, French, and Dutch descent. In the following decades, immigrants came into the mountains from the piedmont and were joined by southern European and black families whose members had been recruited to work in the developing resource industries.

By the mid to late nineteenth century the region had seen the development of a relatively stable agricultural economy and a complex rural society. As historian Ron Eller notes:

Few areas of the United States in the late nineteenth century more closely exemplified Thomas Jefferson's vision for a democratic society than did the agricultural communities of the Southern Appalachians. Long after the death of Jefferson and long after the nation as a whole had turned down the Hamiltonian path toward industrialism, the Southern Appalachian mountains remained a land of small farms and scattered open-country villages. Although traditional patterns of agricultural life persisted in other parts of the nation— in the rural South, the Mid-West, and the more remote sections of the North East—nowhere did the self-sufficient family farm so dominate the culture and social system as it did in the Appalachian South. [Eller 1982, p. 3]

Following the Civil War, the region experienced relative isolation from communication centers and trade, as well as limited availability of revenues for education, roads, and other communication systems. The Civil War had been a time of great internal division in the southern Appalachians. Many counties and families were split as strong Confederacy sentiment ran into conflict with Union and isolationist points of view. Not only was the region ravaged by the battles of the war and families split over the ideological conflicts, but pro-Unionism in the mountains did not go unnoticed by the Confederate factions who controlled the legislative purse-strings of southern states. The states' limited funds would not have stretched far into the mountains anyway, given the high cost of road building, for example, but resentment of mountain pro-Unionism virtually precluded spending for mountain roads and schools.

During the 1880s, there was a major "discovery" of Appalachia by the local color writers and journalists of the day, who saw much in the region to entertain and amuse the American public. The region was described initially in terms of romantic wonder. But, by the 1890s, this wonder had become distress about the imagined degradation and degeneracy observed in the mountains. These writers found an Appalachia disenfranchised by the ravages of the Civil War and spent what brief time they devoted to the area describing illiteracy, isolation, and subsistence living. Mountain people were viewed as hopeless but proud, desperate but industrious. The descriptions emerging from this period are rife with contradictions and both positive and negative extremes. The people of the mountains are seen as noble, first-generation frontiersmen yet degenerate, and this image has grown to be perceived as fact through American fiction.

The northern Protestant denominations, following the local color writers, established mission fields in the region. They saw the region as "unchurched," since their denominations were not represented there. In addition, the new mission churches saw in Appalachia no sense of community, as defined by the presence of churches and schools (Shapiro 1978) and, seeing this need, envisioned that they could create community by giving to the people of the region what they were lacking, that is, churches and schools. They thus saw their mission to be one of uplifting the region through these two institutions.

Several hundred denominational and a dozen "independent" schools were established during this time, and from this effort emerged the institutionalization of Appalachian "otherness" (Shapiro

1978). The churches, following the local color writers, saw the region as a "social problem." They relied heavily on the local color writers' insights and, as a matter of fact, used Mary Noailles Murfree's *In the Tennessee Mountains* as a text (Shapiro 1978).

Meanwhile, the resources of the region were discovered by developing industrial interests outside the region. Speculation in minerals and timberlands, begun much earlier in the region's history, intensified during this period. Around the turn of the century the railroads opened up the mountains to commerce in a major way, and the industrial appetites of the rapidly industrializing society began gnawing at the natural resources of the region. At the same time as coal and land agents appeared in rural farm communities in central Appalachia with offers to purchase mineral rights from farmers whose livelihood was precarious, the availability of a cheap labor force began attracting manufacturing interests to the mountain fringe area. Between 1900 and 1930, 600 company towns sprang up in the southern Appalachians, drawing mountain families from the farm and into factory towns (Eller 1978).

Acquisition of coal lands by outside corporations meant outside control of local communities and local services and, ultimately, local political processes. For example, "through land acquisitions of the early 1900's, a very near majority of Harlan County [Kentucky] has fallen into the hands of absentee owners" (Childers 1979, p. 86). The Appalachian Land Ownership Task Force "found ownership of land and minerals in rural Appalachia to be highly concentrated among a few absentee and corporate owners, resulting in little land actually being available to local people" (1979, p. 1). For Mingo County, West Virginia, and other coal rich counties in central Appalachia, "Out-of-state corporations whose prime concern has been to extract the mineral wealth at the lowest cost to themselves, often leave in the wake of their profit a landless people, staggering death and injury toll in the mines, environment in ruin, and particularly low property tax revenues to county governments" (County Mirrors Appalachian Patterns, 1979, p. 106).

Absentee landownership has also been the result of a growing emphasis on tourism in Appalachia. Resort land speculation and development began to a limited degree during the nineteenth and early twentieth centuries in exclusive areas like Flat Rock, Roan Mountain, Blowing Rock, and Linville, North Carolina. During the 1960s, the mountains witnessed the rapid acceleration of land speculation and the development of a full-scale tourist industry. With the new development, land prices began skyrocketing. With the increase in land values and land taxes, farm families have been forced to sell land and/ or seek employment in the resort and related industries. Likewise, the cost of food and other commodities has risen locally, reflecting the influx of the wealthy tourist market, so that resort areas have become expensive places to live. The taxes and cost of living make it difficult for the small farm to survive, and young families are often precluded from buying land at all. The resort industry is characterized by low-wage, seasonal employment, with frequent layoffs reflecting seasonal demands, and frequent slack cycles caused by gas shortages and the weather. Although the rural family finds less and less support from the land and increasing dependence on public work, work in resort-related enterprises is at best unpredictable.

The growth of the tourist industry in Appalachia has been due in part to the concentration of landownership by the federal government. The U.S. Forest Service is the largest single owner of Appalachian lands, with control of well over 5 million acres of land in the six states of Georgia, Kentucky, North Carolina, Tennessee, Virginia, and West Virginia (Kahn 1978). It has been pointed out that federal ownership of land means lost property tax revenues to local counties and higher tax rates for local owners, limits on productive capacity and development potential, outside manipulation of timber revenues, and high poverty rates (Kahn 1978; Efird 1979).

While a wide range of agencies and organizations have been active in the Appalachian region, the unique factors of regional history, discovery, and interpretation have helped to shape the approaches taken to addressing regional problems. David Whisnant has summarized the point of view of selected missionary, planning, and development agencies as follows:

1. They generally assume that Appalachia is a "deviant subculture" whose problems owe more to physical isolation, depleted gene pools, pathological inbreeding, clan wars, hookworm, moonshining, and welfarism than to the nation's unceasing demands on the region for cheap labor, land, raw materials, and energy.

2. Like the missionaries who insisted that mountain children would be saved only if they learned which side the fork goes on, the plans and programs have insisted that their grandchildren mold themselves to bureaucratic conceptions of middle-class social organization and lifeways.

3. They accept mainstream values and idealized social, economic, and political norms as the natural boundary of feasible approaches to development.

4. They reject any approach to planned, democratic, community-based

public development that promises to alter—or fails to rationalize—established patterns of private entrepreneurial development. [Whisnant 1980, pp. xix-xx]

FAMILY ROLES IN HISTORICAL CONTEXT

Prior to the industrialization of the region, which came quite late in areas like western North Carolina, agriculture and a barter economy were basic factors influencing social life. The settlers established largely self-sufficient homesteads in which each nuclear family was a total production and consumption unit with a clearly defined, yet flexible, division of labor based on age and sex. Whereas individual families were the basic economic units, groups of families came together frequently for large-scale cooperative work activities, for sharing special times in individual and family life cycles such as marriages and births, and in times of community or individual crisis such as illness, injury, or death.

While various writers around the turn of the century comment on the lack of community in the mountains, evidenced by the absence of central churches and schools, others eloquently describe the community of mountain folks based on shared history, belief, experiences, work, trials, and joys. Emma Bell Miles (1975) tells us there is no community of mountaineers in outsider's terms, yet the people are linked to each other as individuals and as friends.

Many observers have described the rural mountain family as simply patriarchal with some exceptions. However, a more useful way of looking at sex roles—and one that explains more facets of life—is to view power, authority, and influence as separate entities, which different people have in different amounts, for different tasks, and which change as people move through the life cycle.

In the traditional agricultural community, men have greater authority in the public spheres of life, while women have greater power in the domestic sphere (power here being the ability to get things done, as opposed to authority, which is publicly recognized and legitimized rights and responsibilities). For both sexes, middle age is a time of hard work. Men reach the height of their public influence in late middle age. For women, however, middle age is a low point, as children are leaving the home and domination by a husband often reaches its peak. Old age for men is a time of waning influence, as the next generation of men is replacing them in work activities. For women, old age is a time of consolidation of power. Women's domestic work never ceases, yet it eases with age. Further, women's public influence may be achieved indirectly through grown sons or directly through widowhood. In the domestic sphere, women's influence over grown children increases as helping and advising relationships are established with children who are establishing their own families. The old widow, in fact, is totally free for the first time in her life and above rebuke. Emma Bell Miles comments at length on this state of affairs, devoting a chapter to "Grandmother and Sons," and noting that "the best society in the mountains—that is to say, the most interesting—is that of the young married men and that of the older women" (Miles 1975, p. 36).

With industrialization, sex roles began to change in the mountains. The textile industries came into the mountain fringes in the 1930s looking for new sources of cheap labor. Mountain families left the farm for stable work in the hundreds of new textile towns, like Gastonia, Lenoir, and Hickory, North Carolina, and became mill town workers, tied completely to the mill structures. By the 1950s, small mills had moved into the mountains and began hiring women from farm families whose income required buttressing.

The industries hired women, according to the anthropologists Collins and Finn (1976), because women "are willing or perhaps unable to be unwilling to take secondary jobs." The industries are characterized by low wages, poor working conditions, arbitrary discipline, and no career ladders. The local male labor force is simply denied access to these jobs. Many women see their jobs as a temporary solution to a family's economic situation. Union organizing attempts are met with threats of violence or of plant closing. As a union organizer in several small textile plants recently stated, older women are willing to organize but are hampered by fear of violence and fear of plant closings, both based on reality. Younger women are not so enthusiastic, since they see their jobs as temporary solutions to their family's economic problems.

Besides facing double jeopardy in their status as women and as residents of rural areas, Appalachian women also face the burden of a double day; that is, rural women spend more time working inside and outside the home than do their urban counterparts. Women are generally ultimately responsible for home and children whether or not they have outside paid employment.

Through "public work," the traditional women's role in the family and the community is drastically altered. Women gain power in the allocation of household resources and increase their influence over the decisions in the community, particularly in education and health care delivery systems. They are no longer tied to the authority of the once dominant husband in the household and have greater freedom through their roles outside the family, despite their powerlessness in the wider society because of the secondary position of their work.

Mountain families who move off the mountain to factory towns on the mountain fringe face stresses resulting from a new class structure, lack of access to land, and a myriad of problems in adjusting to factory dominated life. At the same time, rural families who stay on the land face different sorts of problems. For the working wife, new income sources and exposure to ideas in the workplace threaten traditional relationships with husbands. While many couples adapt to new work roles with ease, for others, particularly when the husband is unemployed, the new expectations and new freedoms can threaten the relationship. More troublesome for most women, however, is the guilt that comes from having to leave the care and raising of children to others. As mountain women have been raised to have primary responsibility for their children, to leave them with strangers is difficult. Finally, the double day faced by women in the work force throughout the United States is particularly grueling among rural families deriving some products from the land. Women are plagued with fatigue and stress, compounded by guilt and pressure from family.

IMPLICATIONS FOR MENTAL HEALTH SYSTEMS

Implied in this brief overview of the historical development of Appalachia and its impact on family roles is that Appalachia has undergone industrialization in the same way as America at large. Appalachia is not the quaint land represented by the media in such images as James Dickey's *Deliverance* and Al Capp's Li'l Abner. Mountain people have long been integrated into the national economy and have had to cope with a particular mix of urban industrial and rural agrarian ways of life throughout this century. Appalachians maintain many traditional family and community social patterns while experiencing radical sex role changes. They retain a special relationship to the land and to a place while experiencing the new social structure and detachment from the soil accompanying industrialization. It is possible that this mix of urban and rural culture patterns has buffered the otherwise wrenching nature of industrialization in the mountains. Nevertheless, the stress experienced by mountain people in the context of this rapid social change is significant. There is a need to better understand its nature and resolution.

In many ways, Appalachians probably have had to suffer greater stress than other Americans, considering the particular features of development in the mountains. The acquisition and development of mountain land and resources by outside interests has contributed to diminishing control by regional people and local communities over their own environments and economy. This contributes to a strong sense of powerlessness, based on real economic fact. At the same time, given the patronizing and culture-dominating approach of the mainstream society including helping agencies, Appalachians are not particularly receptive to helping professionals. Mental health services in the mountains will have to deal perceptively with the issues of appropriate therapeutic models for and means of delivering services to Appalachian people, if they are to contribute to a reversal of the unfortunate historical pattern of domination and powerlessness in the mountains.

REFERENCES

Appalachian Land Ownership Task Force. 1979. *Land ownership patterns and their impacts on Appalachian communities*. Boone, N.C.: Center for Appalachian Studies, Appalachian State University.

Childers, J. 1979. Absentee ownership of Harlan County. In *A landless people in a rural region: A reader on land ownership and property taxation in Appalachia*, ed. S. Fisher, 81-92. New Market, Tenn.: Highlander Research and Education Center.

Collins, T.W., and C.L. Finn. 1976. Mountain women in a changing labor market. *The Tennessee Anthropologist* 1(2):104-11.

County mirrors Appalachian patterns: Inequities in the tax system. 1979. In *A landless people in a rural region: A reader on land ownership and property taxation in Appalachia*, ed. S. Fisher, 106-107. New Market, Tenn.: Highlander Research and Education Center.

Efird, C. 1979. Public land ownership: Its impact on Swain County, N.C. In *Citizen participation in rural land use planning for the Tennessee Valley*, ed. L. Jones, 62-66. Nashville: Agricultural Marketing Project.

Eller, R. 1978. Industrialization and social change in Appalachia, 1880-1930. In *Colonialism in modern America: The Appalachian case*, ed. H. Lewis, L. Johnson, and D. Askins, 35-46. Boone, N.C.: Appalachian Consortium Press.

Eller, R. 1982. *Miners, millhands, and mountaineers: Industrialization of the Appalachian South, 1880-1930*. Knoxville: University of Tennessee Press.

Kahn, S. 1978. The forest service and Appalachia. In *Colonialism in modern America: The Appalachian case*, ed. H. Lewis, L. Johnson, and D. Askins, 85-109. Boone, N.C.: The Appalachian Consortium Press.

Miles, E.B. 1975. *The spirit of the mountains*. Knoxville: University of Tennessee Press. Originally published New York: Pott, 1905.

Shapiro, H.D. 1978. *Appalachia on our mind: The southern mountains and mountaineers in the American consciousness, 1870-1920*. Chapel Hill: University of North Carolina Press.

Whisnant, D.E. 1980. *Modernizing the mountaineer: People, power, and planning in Appalachia*. New York: Burt Franklin and Co.

2

Appalachian Family Ties

SUSAN EMLEY KEEFE

No ethnography of Appalachians fails to speak of them as familistic. The family is the central unit of rural Appalachian social organization. It is the basis of an individual's identity. In many cases, kinship is described as the only basis for social relationships among rural mountaineers; neighbors and friends in some way always overlap with kin. We know most about rural Appalachian family organization at this point and so this paper is focused on it.

Of course, kinship is the basis for social organization in any society, including mainstream American society in general. However, the meaning of kinship and its structure varies from society to society. Appalachian kinship and mainstream American kinship share many characteristics but there are important differences. In the mental health profession, conceptions of "healthy" family life and appropriate therapies for families with problems tend to be based on the model provided by mainstream American families. This paper addresses the need to take into consideration cultural differences in assessing and treating Appalachian families.

THE APPALACHIAN FAMILY GROUP

The Appalachian concept of family is patterned differently than for mainstream American non-Appalachians who may also live in the region (Keefe, Reck, and Reck 1985). Appalachian natives perceive the category of "family" to include the nuclear family (spouse and children), the family of orientation (parents and brothers and sisters), and generally brothers' and sisters' spouses and children. Typically, the nuclear family is a separate household unit and is the fundamental unit of social organization, but it is not conceived of as an entirely independent unit. Rather than splitting from the family of orientation, new nuclear families are added to the larger family. This family unit, then, is made up of many households. In their work in eastern Kentucky, Schwarzweller, Brown and Mangalam (1971) refer to this as a *family group*.

Frequent visiting and exchange takes place among members of these closely related households, most often between parents and their married children and between siblings who live nearby or feel special affection toward one another. Mutual aid involves both major and minor exchange of goods and services and takes place on a daily basis as well as in times of crisis. Certain kinds of aid tend to be associated exclusively with the family group. At marriage, for example, parents may provide the newlyweds with land to accommodate housing. This can result in the frequently observed rural Appalachian settlement pattern of a main house with adjacent trailers or secondary houses occupied by married children. Sometimes parents may also allow newlyweds to move into their household temporarily, usually for less than a year. Elderly parents may have children or grandchildren come by to help them with chores and farm work.

The family group may also be the decision-making unit. The family as a whole discusses local events, forms opinions, and arrives at a consensus based on group discussion. The family also acts as a social control agent regarding deviant behavior. Though the group will almost always support members against outsiders, it will also apply criticism, gossip, and ridicule to keep members in line.

Finally, the family group is the emotional support unit. The family shares common values and ideals and provides members with a sense of belonging, affection, and security. Family members know they have a group that can be counted on for help in times of crisis.

Let me give an example of a close-knit Appalachian family. When I first knew this family, it consisted of my informant (Mrs. D), her elderly mother, her aunt (mother's sister), her three unmarried children, two older children and their families, and her nephew and his son. The members of this family group are concentrated in two towns about 15 miles apart. Not only do the kin in this group visit back and forth frequently (mostly without formally scheduled visits), they also help each other out with housework, gifts of food, and sometimes very expensive gifts (for example, Mrs. D's well-to-do aunt gave each of Mrs. D's two youngest sons a new car after they graduated from high school). The young people move somewhat freely from one household to the other. My informant's two youngest sons have lived at one time or another with their great aunt, and my informant's nephew often moves in with her for long periods of time. Recently, he went to stay with his grandmother for several days because he felt she was becoming increasingly ill. My informant's Christmas stockings are an indication of her family, all of whom gather together at her home on Christmas day; she has a stocking for each person in the family group hung on her stairway bannister, a total of 16 stockings.

Other relatives are perceived by native Appalachians as falling into two groups: (1) relatives/kin, who include more distantly related blood kin and their spouses (such as grandparents, aunts, uncles, and cousins); and (2) spouse's kin. Relatives can be a large group but typically informants do not recognize kin beyond the grandparents' ascending generation, grandchildrens' descending generation, and first cousins in their own generation. "Relatives" see each other and exchange goods and services less frequently than "family." They most often come together at weddings, funerals, and reunions. Spouse's kin are not conceived of as the informant's relatives or kin. Rather, they are referred to as "my wife's family" or "my husband's family." Visiting is less frequent with spouse's kin than with the informant's own family. Sometimes this results in interesting visiting patterns within the nuclear family. One woman I interviewed, for example, married into her husband's community. One of his brothers lives nearby and the brothers visit daily, often at her house. However, she says, she doesn't really talk to her brother-in-law. Her concern is directed more toward her own "family," particularly her parents with whom she visits every Sunday.

THE KINDRED

For Appalachians, then, blood relatives are set definitely apart from and are perceived as more significant than in-laws. Anthropologists refer to the network of blood kin traced through both sides of the family (father's and mother's) as a kindred. Typically, kindreds are considered to be noncorporate because of the overlapping nature of group membership and consequent lack of structural boundaries. For example, in a nuclear family the father's kindred would not include his in-laws (i.e., the mother's kindred), while their son's kindred would include both sets of relatives. Kindred membership thus varies depending on the individual anchoring the kindred. Lack of boundedness results in the kindred having few functions as a formal group, for example, as a landowning unit or a political faction. On the other hand, kindreds can function as flexible and adaptive kin networks forming the basis for socializing and mutual aid. As such, kindreds are the basis for kinship in mainstream America.

In Appalachia, however, the kindred appears to function differently. Here the kindred is much more of a bounded or corporate group. Caroline Bryant in *We're All Kin* (1981) describes kin groups in the eastern Tennessee community she studied as "quasi-descent groups," which trace relations back to a single ancestor. These groups come together formally at family reunions but otherwise tend to act more informally as networks of information and support.

Family reunions are for people who trace their descent back to a particular ancestor, usually a man but sometimes a married couple. The reunion is the one big, planned social effort for the kindred and is sometimes attended by several hundred people. It is generally held outdoors in the summer on the home church grounds, at a public meeting place such as a school, or at the "homeplace" or family farm. The local family members bring the "covered dishes" and prepare food for all. After dinner, there may be groups of singers who perform, preaching by several people, and even public addresses by political figures. Often a prize or recognition is given to the person who came the greatest distance to the reunion, to the oldest and the youngest family members attending, and to those celebrating some special occasion, such as graduation or a birthday. There may also be recreational activities such as a softball game. The reunion, then, is the one consistent social event for the kindred and is important for reaffirming the group's identity and social contacts of members. Most individuals have the opportunity to attend one or more reunions during the year. Family reunions, of course, are not unique to southern Appalachia, but they tend to be found mainly in other rural areas of the country, such as the Midwest, where kinship is more significant than in urban communities (see Ayoub 1966).

Although it varies, the reunion tends to emphasize the kindred members, that is, those tied by blood. Spouses of kindred members may not feel a part of the proceedings. In fact, one woman I interviewed told me she did not go to her husband's family reunion because "they don't want me." But in the small community she studied, Bryant (1981) found that in-laws are not set apart so much; instead, the similarities are stressed ("we're all kin"). This may be more true of small, isolated, homogeneous communities where conflict and differences are perceived as more threatening.

Typically, an individual goes to only one family reunion; in other words, the individual *chooses* a line with which to affiliate. Thus, it is important to emphasize that kin groups in Appalachia are to a great extent voluntary groups. One can choose a segment of the family with which to ally. Kinship is also voluntary in that people often choose not to recognize others as kin, which may happen, for example, if there has been conflict with another in the family. This can result in kin factions that ultimately form two distinct kin groups. Kin group divisions can also come about when relatives settle at a distance from one another. For example, one family surname group in the county we studied are all descendants of three brothers who settled in three areas of the county in the 18th century; yet, the descendants generally do not recognize this relationship, claiming to be unrelated or so distantly related that it is insignificant. Kinship in this family is claimed only with those living close by.

While the kindred in one sense is a voluntary group, in another sense it is not. Members generally do not *think* of the larger family as a voluntary unit but one ascribed by blood. In other words, once having made the choice to affiliate with one line, the individual is bound by certain strictures to that group. For one thing, an individual has a number of obligations and rights or benefits as a result of belonging to a kindred:

1. Jobs are acquired through kin: for example, school authorities often hire family in the community; elected officials may appoint kin.

2. Personal and group identity are based primarily on the family. A person is first a member of a family and then has other identities, such as age, sex, or vocation. The community judges a person's character by reference to his or her kin ties. If your family has a reputation for honesty, for example, you are assumed to be honest.

Furthermore, in rural Appalachia, family and community are often coterminous. Families tend to be identified with a particular part of the county and local identity, which is sometimes referred to by Appalachian scholars as "association with place," and the place is thus bound up with family ties. The association of family and community becomes tangible in such things as land inheritance, the homeplace, and the family cemetery.

3. Kin are "loyal" to one another, which includes moral and economic overtones. Kin owe respect and honesty to kin. They will not cheat them financially and will usually give them a better deal in buying things, such as land or cars. They help each other out in cooperative labor projects and mutual aid.

4. Political support is expected between kin. Kin vote for kin, and they do not run against kinfolk.

5. Kin provide emotional and moral support for each other. They support each other when challenged by outsiders. They give comfort in times of trouble (adapted from Hicks 1976).

These obligations and benefits demonstrate why kinship is so important in Appalachian communities; kinship is intertwined with all aspects of life: political, economic, social, and moral.

Where the kindred is significant, as in Appalachia, we tend to find the cousin relationship important. First cousins especially tend to be close kin. In her study of a small, relatively isolated Tennessee community, Elmora Matthews (1965) finds the naming of children, for example, follows collateral ties to cousins and siblings rather than to parents or grandparents. She finds more friendships between cousins and siblings than between any other kin, too. Individuals often marry cousins, including first cousins, which strengthens the already strong ties between collateral kin. Matthews also finds the phenomenon of "double cousins" common in her community. Double cousins are the children of siblings who married siblings. Siblings and their double cousins are the only individuals in the kinship system who share exactly the same kindred. Being related to each other by "double bonds," through both parents, further heightens the significance of the kin tie.

The pattern of family ties I have been describing, which I have identified as Appalachian, is associated with rural residence and geographic stability. It does not appear to vary with socioeconomic status in rural areas. There are indications, however, that urban middle class Appalachians are more likely to follow the mainstream American pattern.

CONTRAST WITH MAINSTREAM AMERICANS

Among non-Appalachian mainstream Americans, the most basic social unit is the nuclear family, made up of parents and children (Keefe, Reck, and Reck 1985). The nuclear family is perceived as an independent unit, and frequently this is reinforced by geographic isolation from other kin. A second category of kin, many times perceived as closely connected to the nuclear family, is referred to as family/relatives/kin. These have "close" family ties; as one informant put it, these relatives are "those who really care about you." This group typically includes parents, brothers and sisters and their spouses and children. It may also include grandparents, aunts, uncles, cousins, and spouse's kin. It is these relatives with whom exchange and visiting take place. A third category of kin is identified as relatives/distant relatives and includes blood kin and spouse's kin not included in the second type. These relatives are seen infrequently and rarely participate in the exchange of goods and services.

Thus, mainstream Americans tend not to make the same sharp distinction between the kindred and in-laws as do Appalachians. Mainstream Americans have a more flexible system of kin definition; there is more choice available in the designation of those who are considered close kin and those who are not (for example, a favorite aunt may be included, an obnoxious cousin may be left out). In-laws often are considered significant kin and may be important emotional supports. Of course, this also means that mainstream Americans have less-corporate kindreds and although, therefore, kin are less demanding, they are also less helpful.

Another basic reason that kinfolk are less helpful for mainstream Americans is the lack of geographic proximity. Mainstream Americans define a group of close kin who are the extended family members they can count on for help. They provide the family identity for individuals. They are the relatives who are worried about and talked about most. And they are the kin who provide family members with a psychological feeling of well-being stemming from their support of the individual. But they may be seen only occasionally, during holidays and vacations and in times of crisis, due to the widespread residence pattern of mainstream American extended families (Keefe 1984).

Appalachians, on the other hand, have a kin group that is geographically proximate. In fact, kin may all be located within a particular hollow or community. The often heard "Everybody around here is kin" may be literally true. This means kin are visited frequently, often daily. The ties of kinship tend to overlap with friends, neighbors, coworkers, church members, and so on, creating dense social networks. Close proximity also allows mutual aid to take place in day-to-day affairs as well as in times of crisis. Small exchanges of food, baby clothes, personal advice, and so forth, go on daily. There is exchange of labor. Cooperative activities can be crucial for farmers who rely on it to fix barns, butcher hogs, and harvest tobacco. Nursing care is provided in times of sickness. Wives help out when babies are born. Orphaned children are taken in by the rest of the family. This geographic proximity ensures the continuity and strength of the Appalachian kin group.

FAMILY TIES AND STRESS

Strong extended family ties are often characterized in the mental health literature as having one of two outcomes. Some authors emphasize that the extended family structure of many ethnic groups promotes mental health by providing security, stability, identity, and emotional support in times of need (Jaco 1960; Madsen 1969). Other authors argue that strong family ties prevent individual growth and development by fostering dependency and inhibiting the development of achievement motivation and socioeconomic mobility (Group for the Advancement of Psychiatry, Committee on the Family 1970; Weller 1965). Let me take a moment here to consider some of the mental health outcomes of kinship ties in southern Appalachia.

As noted earlier, rural families in Appalachia tend to be clustered in particular geographic areas according to historical settlement patterns and claims to original land grants. Many roads, valleys, and hollows are named after the family group that predominates in the area. Thus, family and community often merge, strengthening social ties and identity. In most cases, this has a positive effect on individuals. Some families, however, have reputations that may be characterized unfavorably. In each school district the Recks and I studied, for example, a few local surnames tend to be associated with lower-class background and poor success in school. Children entering school with these surnames are automatically labeled potential dropouts and are treated differently throughout their school years. Not surprisingly, almost all of these youths do in fact drop out. One family suffers from the reputation of their relatively isolated community, which is named after their surname. This community has had several colorful characters and violent disturbances since the turn of the century and has become notorious in the county. As a result, individuals with this family surname are stigmatized in any social encounter. In these cases, family surname functions as effectively as physical or racial traits in ascribing lower class status.

Strong family ties, of course, are reinforced by strong, positive emotional ties. Clearly, these are important to the formation and maintenance of a strong identity, a feeling of "roots," and pride in one's heritage. Ties beyond the nuclear family provide real support and reciprocal aid. At the same time, the strength of family ties can have stressful outcomes. David Looff (1971), for example, points out that school phobia has been a common problem in Appalachia, because of the exaggerated dependency of some young children. Furthermore, where parents and siblings are highly significant emotionally, problems and conflicts in the family group or death of a family member may cause as much stress for an adult as conflict with or the death of a spouse. One woman I interviewed, for example, was deeply affected by her closest brother's death. She had stayed with him for seven and one-half weeks while he lay dying in the hospital. She talked about him frequently during the interviews and remarked "I haven't been well since he died." This woman is very close to her mother, who has also been hit hard by her son's death, and they share their grief. What is suggested here is that the causes of stress and such instruments as the Life Stress Scale (Gunderson and Rahe 1974) are culture bound.

It is clear that strong family ties per se are not inherently beneficial or unbeneficial to individuals. In fact, they may serve both to promote mental health and cause stress, something true of any form of family organization. What must be determined is the impact of the particular form of family organization on various types and on the severity of emotional problems. Furthermore, it is essential to evaluate the way in which family organization varies within an ethnic group by socioeconomic class and rural or urban residence. Appalachian family organization as just described best fits rural mountain residents. Urban middle class Appalachians are quite likely to operate within more mainstreamlike families and might be expected to differ little from non-Appalachians in the experience of family-related emotional problems.

Close family ties can become stressful when there is conflict among kin. And most ethnographers note that despite the emphasis on strong kin ties in Appalachia, there is also a great deal of conflict within kin groups. Frequently, these are between siblings' families and they may be due to competing relationships introduced by spouses or to conflict over inheritance after the parents' death.

As an example, Mrs. D, cited previously, has one sister who leads a life-style she disapproves of and with whom she has never felt close, although they visit frequently. In the last year, coinciding with the illness and death of their mother, their relationship has grown increasingly strained. Part of the strain was due to Mrs. D's accusation that her sister's son had succeeded in getting their mother to sign over her house to him at a time when she was not legally competent to do so. This is now being fought in the courts, and combined with her mother's death, it has caused Mrs. D considerable emotional stress. It has also created factions within the kindred, as members have been forced to choose sides on the issue.

It is important to recognize, then, that close family ties do not ensure social harmony. Rather, they imply that when social conflict occurs, it is likely to involve kin with whom most significant interactions take place.

IMPLICATIONS FOR INTERVENTION

There are important implications here for mental health services and other agencies. First, conceptions of the "healthy" family are culture based. When Jack Weller (1965), for example, criticizes rural Appalachian couples for not talking to each other more, the criticism is based on the middle-class mainstream American expectation that husbands and wives socialize as a couple with other couples and have common friends and interests. The rural Appalachian norm, on the other hand, is one of gender-specific roles and social groups. As another example, the expectation that adult children for the most part should be independent of their parents applies to middle-class mainstream Americans; in rural Appalachia, children are expected to listen to and follow their parents' counsel for life.

Just as health is culturally defined, so are stress and illness. In rural Appalachia, where close family ties are the norm, people feel great stress if they do *not* have a close kindred to rely on and give them support. In the earlier example, one of the most distressing things for Mrs. D concerning the recent friction in her family is the loss of family unity. This was particularly true at Christmas time, when she chose not to hold the traditional family gathering.

Another source of stress for Appalachians stems from acculturation and change in identification as urbanization and the in-migration of newcomers touch the lives of rural residents in the region. Appalachian families have always had to deal with the effects of out-migration of family members. With increasing migration to cities within the mountains, Appalachians who stay in the region now also feel the loss of the traditional extended family and this can be stressful. Furthermore, with the arrival in the mountains of people from outside the region, who come armed with the stereotypes and derogatory names associated with Appalachia, natives of the region must continually reassess their identity and attempt to reaffirm it in a positive way. Societies in the process of rapid change produce great stress and a greater likelihood of mental illness. We must become sensitive to the ways in which social change is involved in causing individuals' feelings of stress in the mountains.

Treatment must also be culturally relevant. One of my students in doing an internship in an Appalachian mental health agency found that one of the stated priorities in dealing with clients had to do with housing. High on the list of preferred housing arrangements was living alone, while living with family was not preferred. This concept of preferred living arrangements has little to do with mental health per se and everything to do with normal and acceptable living arrangements in mainstream America, where one should not be "sponging" off one's parents after the age of eighteen.

In addition to recognizing and working to reinforce rather than negate important cultural traits, I think it is imperative to formulate mental health services with Appalachian culture in mind. Given the kin-based nature of Appalachian society, one of the ways in which this could be accomplished is to begin with the family (and not necessarily the nuclear family) as the basic unit for health care rather than the individual. For example, family members' support and endorsement of therapeutic care may be indispensible for treatment. If family members are not acknowledged and consulted, they may intervene and prevent successful continuation of treatment. Second, therapies that work with larger social units, such as family network therapy, are probably very appropriate in Appalachia.

Finally, let me reiterate the need to identify the cultural background of clients. We cannot assume that Appalachians are similar to non-Appalachians, nor can we assume that all Appalachians are alike. Therapists need to know something about the client's birthplace, migration history, socioeconomic class, and rural or urban background. Along with this, it would be important to get information on family structure, to see if it fits the cultural norm and where the sources of support and stress might be. Furthermore, future research must investigate the heterogeneity of Appalachian life in order to determine more precisely the nature and the variety in form of the Appalachian family.

NOTES

This research was funded by the National Science Foundation, grant no. BNS-8218234. Much of what I have to say on family has emerged from research done with

Gregory Reck and Mae Reck on ethnicity and education in a county in western North Carolina.

REFERENCES

Ayoub, M. 1966. The family reunion. *Ethnology* 5:415-33.

Bryant, F.C. 1981. *We're all kin: A cultural study of a mountain neighborhood.* Knoxville: University of Tennessee Press.

Group for the Advancement of Psychiatry, Committee on the Family. 1970. Integration and mal-integration in Spanish-American family patterns. In *Treatment of families in conflict: The clinical study of family process.* New York: Jason Arsonson.

Gunderson, E.K.E., and R.H. Rahe, eds. 1974. *Life stress and illness.* Springfield, Ill.: Charles C Thomas.

Hicks, G.L. 1976. *Appalachian valley.* New York: Holt, Rinehart and Winston.

Jaco, E.G. 1960. *The social epidemiology of mental disorders: A psychiatric survey of Texas.* New York: Russell Sage Foundation.

Keefe, S.E. 1984. Real and ideal extended familism among Mexican Americans and Anglo Americans: On the meaning of "close" family ties. *Human Organization* 43:65-70.

Keefe, S.E., U.M.L. Reck, and G.G. Reck. 1985. Family and education in southern Appalachia. Paper presented at the annual meeting of the Appalachian Studies Conference, Berea, Ky.

Looff, D.H. 1971. *Appalachia's children: The challenge of mental health.* Lexington: University Press of Kentucky.

Madsen, W. 1969. Mexican-Americans and Anglo-Americans: A comparative study of mental health in Texas. In *Changing perspectives in mental illness,* eds. S.C. Plog and R.B. Edgerton, 217-41. New York: Holt, Rinehart and Winston.

Matthews, E.M. 1965. *Neighbor and kin: Life in a Tennessee ridge community.* Nashville: Vanderbilt University Press.

Schwarzweller, H.K., J.S. Brown, and J.J. Mangalam. 1971. *Mountain families in transition: A case study of Appalachian migration.* University Park, Pa.: Pennsylvania State University Press.

Weller, J.E. 1965. *Yesterday's people: Life in contemporary Appalachia.* Lexington: University Press of Kentucky.

3

Religion in Southern Appalachia

RICHARD A. HUMPHREY

Quite commonly, religion in Appalachia is greatly misunderstood or misrepresented. The traditional religion of Appalachia has been under attack since the 1880s by missionaries, teachers, and mainstream America through the mass media and state and federal agencies and programs. Mental health professionals have not been an exception to the rule. For the most part, psychologists as well as missionaries and teachers have not seriously attempted to understand the southern Appalachian people's religion. This is all the more unfortunate considering that the one aspect on which scholars, social workers, and the Appalachian people generally agree is that Appalachian religion today is one of the most traditional social institutions in the region and the one institution that has steadfastly resisted change. And, as Loyal Jones points out, the fact is that "One has to understand the religion of the mountaineer before he can begin to understand mountaineers" (in Mauer 1974, p. 107).

Little understanding has been forthcoming, however. Instead, for more than a century, mountain people have had the "do-gooder from off" tell them what is wrong with them. This perspective, combined with the "culture of poverty theory" of the 1960s in which mountaineers have been called yesterday's people, has made Appalachian residents suspicious, even hostile, to the social worker. John Fetterman, in his book *Stinking Creek*, states it very forcefully, "The mountaineer would like to have one person—one day—come into his hollow and show some signs of approval of the way he has lived over the decades, and the way he wants to live forever, and not try to change him without first knowing him" (1967, p. 33).

In order to gain insight concerning mountaineer's religious behavior and its impact on mental health and associated services, we need first to look at the manner in which religion developed in this area and then to examine how religion aids or hinders the mental health professional in fulfilling necessary tasks in the region.

HISTORICAL PERSPECTIVE

When the first Europeans began to enter southern Appalachia through the Shenandoah Valley in 1730-1750, the family was the only social institution. Soon afterward these families began to establish churches. The family churches developed indigenously in the region, with the exception of churches of German origin and the Scotch-Irish Presbyterians. Generally speaking, there was no established religion in the sense of organized churches or clergy to guide the people. In fact, the region in this period and until the American Revolution had been characterized as ignorant of religion. This judgment should be questioned, however, because the people did have a strong family religion. That is, even though the people had no organized churches or educated clergy, they kept their religion alive in their homes and community through study of the Bible, teaching the religion of their homeland, and through their religious folk traditions. When churches were later established in a community, the extended families in that community formed their foundations.

This indigenous religion was given impetus by the Great Revival that started on the Kentucky frontier and spread back through the mountains in the late 1790s and first decade of the nineteenth century (Boles 1972). This Great Revival of the early nineteenth century, though shared with the rest of the nation, was to leave an indelible imprint on the religion of southern Appalachia. In Appalachia, the revival found no settled religious tradition with which to anchor itself. Even today, many church congregations have not moved far from the frontier religion of that Great Revival.

The revival introduced a very personal, conversion-oriented theology into Appalachia. One became a Christian not by having correct doctrine but by attesting to one's conversion experience. Mountain preaching was now viewed positively if it was exhortative and brought one to conversion. Along with the new ideology and way of preaching, this revival introduced the camp meeting, song schools, gospel songs, shaped-note singing, the mourners' pit, and an emotional religious setting in which revivals were more likely to happen. A revival could take place in any religious service when one or more of these elements were present, whether the religious setting was a sacramental meeting, regular worship, homecoming, memorial or funeral service, or conference or association meeting.

One fascinating example of this evangelical influence on religious settings can be seen at the annual communion services of Union, Regular, United, Separate, Free Will, Christian Unity, and Primitive Baptist churches. An onlooker at one of these services, today, might be reminded of the sacramental meetings held on the Gasper River in 1798. In Appalachia, where the emphasis is not on sacraments as dispensing grace, the traditional churches emphasize biblical ordinances. Elder Willie Hamm, a Union Baptist preacher for the past sixty-two years, gives a description of a biblical ordinance: "We oughten to vary from the teachings of Jesus. If Jesus did it and he told his disciples to do it, then you and I had better do it" (personal interview, June 9, 1977).

Traditional churches in the region practice two or three, or as many as seven, ordinances, including the Southern Baptists' practice of baptism by immersion and the Lord's supper. Some southern Baptists also practice foot washing after communion in accordance with the Gospel of John, as do the Separate, Regular, United Primitive, Free Will, Union, General, Christian Unity, Double Seed Predestinarian, and Duck River Baptists as well as others. In addition, the Primitive Advent Christian, Mennonite, Church of the Brethren, some Methodist churches, and Church of God, and other Holiness-Pentecostal churches also wash feet.

Members of these Appalachian churches tend to be conservative Calvinist in their theology. They see a person, at best, as a forgiven sinner. They believe we are caught in original sin and are only forgiven by the grace of God working in us. Many controversies and church schisms have resulted from differing interpretations of predestination, free will, grace, and salvation. The biblical plan of salvation is taken very seriously and each individual must work it out on his or her own. It is precisely on this theological point that I find Pat Beaver's (1976) "egalitarian ethic" most rigidly at work in the region.[1] According to this theological point of view, we all have one common denominator: we are all sinners who need the mercy of God through His son Jesus Christ to save us from our bondage to sin. The family, their religion, and the Bible are the common heritage of the people, and each one emphasizes the importance of the individual while proclaiming his or her dependence upon family and God for security, relationships, and eternal life. The influence of the Great Revival, the emphasis on biblical ordinances, and a Calvinist theology were permanently implanted in Appalachian culture by the Civil War and the period of cultural and political isolation that followed the war.

A key figure in local areas during this period was the homegrown but unlettered preacher. He helped the people understand their suffering and, with his congregation and the use of church discipline, attempted to preserve the culture of their forebears. This folk preacher did his job so well that revivalism and the emphasis on biblical ordinances became an indigenous part of the religion and the culture. The preacher constantly reminded people of Jesus' words in Matthew 28, where they were called to baptize, make disciples, and maintain the tradition until Jesus came again. He also exhorted them with I Corinthians 11, in which the apostle Paul called them to be imitators of Christ and to maintain the traditions "even as I have delivered them to you." Significantly, unlike the minister of a mainstream Christian church, the preacher in a traditional church in southern Appalachia is not seen as a counselor or problem solver. His primary role is to preach for conviction and conversion. He may provide transportation, financial assistance, and sympathy, but rarely does he give advice or counsel on personal or family problems.

The Bible for most Appalachian churches is "the only rule of faith and practice." Each individual within the fellowship must work out his or her salvation with "fear and trembling." Many mountain people would stress two practices that really separate the traditional mountain Christian from mainline American churches. First, the old-time religion requires baptism in a river or stream, not in "bath tubs" or by sprinkling or pouring, in the same way that Jesus was baptized in the River Jordan. Second, all "old-timey" church congregations wash feet. Some also emphasize the following ordinances: praying for and anointing the sick, marriage, veiling women, the Lord's supper, and the flower service. Further, mountaineers point out that real mountain churches have annual memorial services. They practice church discipline (referred to as being churched), which involves action decided upon by the elders and taken against an individual who is deemed to have violated proprieties of the faith and the church. They have the kiss of peace or a greeting after the service by all members. Their regular Sunday worship also differs from mainstream American churches. They may not meet as often (usually one Saturday and one Sunday or sometimes two Sundays a month), but they meet for a longer period, from three to six hours.

By 1890, southern Appalachian religion had two major emphases: (1) the evangelical or revival focus; and (2) the biblical ordinances, or religion of Zion. Most churches put an emphasis on both. Exceptions are the Primitive Baptists and a few others who affirm the religion of Zion but are against revivals and other "man-made institutions," such as Sunday schools, missionary societies, and musical instruments used in worship.

From the 1880s until World War I, the major challenge in Appalachia came from the churches of mainstream America. Each major denomination, in the North and South, discovered an open mission field in Appalachia. The northern denominations focused on schools and health care facilities. The southern denominations' major emphasis was on evangelism (Hooker 1933). The Baptists and Methodists made the greatest gains in church membership. In fact, over 60% of the churches in Appalachia are either Methodist or Baptist today (Ford 1962). Many of these are still very traditional in their understanding and practice of religion. A rule of thumb is: the further away from the county seat or a city, the more traditional the religious faith and practice will be. On the other hand, the closer to the county seat or a city, the more local churches tend to be like mainstream American churches.

During this later period, the Holiness-Pentecostalist movement, known as the Later Rain Movement, began in Monroe County, Tennessee, and Cherokee County, North Carolina (Conn 1977). This movement, through the various churches of God and other Holiness-Pentecostal churches, is the logical extreme of the religion of Zion. They take the spiritual gifts, especially of I Corinthians 12 and 14, as biblical ordinances.

Since the 1880s southern Appalachia has not only been challenged by mainstream American church missionaries and by the Holiness-Pentecostal movement, but also discovered and literally invaded by the lumber, coal, and tourist industries. The region also became a topic for interpretation by the mass media and the novelist.

Both world wars took many of the young men away from the region. In addition, World War II started the great out-migration of three million persons from Appalachia. This caused a tremendous drain on the traditional mountain religion and culture. When the National Forest Service, Park Service, TVA, and most recently the Appalachian Regional Commission are added to the outside influences that have come into the region in recent decades, one can begin to see why many people of Appalachia are afraid, confused, and even hostile toward outside innovation. No one can really know the influence radio and television has had. However, it also undoubtedly challenges many of the beliefs and practices of the traditional mountaineer and causes difficulties between the generations in a family.

TRADITIONAL RELIGION AND THE
MENTAL HEALTH PROFESSIONAL

From the preceding historical perspective, one should not be surprised at the traditional southern Appalachians' response to mental health programs from the outside. In order to cope with rapid change, the mountaineer turns to the family and religion for security and as an anchor for identity. The mountain church, with its emphasis on the Bible as the "only rule of faith and practice," gives the mountaineer a pattern by which to guide his or her life. Tedra Harmon, of *Fox Fire* renown, stated it plainly one day in his workshop while he crafted a banjo: "The Bible is my map. It shows me the roads, the paths, the valleys, the mountains, the hollers, the people, the sins, and the troubles. But most important of all, it shows me the way to the end of the road and how to live to get there. Without the Bible, a man is lost. No preacher, church, or anybody else can plot my path—I have to" (personal interview, November 5, 1976).

Accordingly, the members of traditional Appalachian churches know that the Bible teaches first to seek the kingdom of God and all else will be added to it. They also know that God calls them to take care of their own. The Bible tells them to take care of the poor, the sick, the hungry, the orphaned, and the widowed, to visit those in prison, and to welcome the stranger. The Bible also tells them to settle their problems outside of the courts. Some have interpreted this as the right to take the law into their own hands, and the news media has brought notoriety to some mountaineers' feuds and violence. To curtail such tendencies, the mountain preacher has an arsenal of scriptural texts warning about "being slow of speech and anger"; about "putting away filthy and loose talk"; about gossiping; about "showing partiality between rich and poor"; about "not judging—especially those outside the church"; about "avoiding stupid and senseless controversy." Then, the preacher reminds his congregation to "correct opponents with gentleness," to "pay their debts," and to "comfort one another because love covers a multitude of sins."[2]

Hence, Appalachian people rebuild barns and houses as an act of Christian love and kindness, if flood or fire destroys them. Children born out of wedlock are often treated and loved as other children. Retarded children are referred to as special gifts of God and are called "blest-born." It is still not uncommon in Appalachia to have three, often four, generations living in one home or one place. The mountaineers' attitude toward welfare is represented by this statement of Bunie Hicks of Beech Creek, North Carolina: "We had slaves once in this nation. I will not be a federal slave" (personal interview, November 6, 1976). Accordingly, in Watauga County, North Carolina, for example, only one-third of the people who are eligible for food stamps apply for them.

The people in southern Appalachia are not only suspicious of the outsider who says he or she is coming to help them but many of them believe that the Bible teaches them to do God's business first. God's business is to get saved and then to take care of their own. According to traditional Appalachian beliefs, social and political issues have no place in the church, and the church members should personally, as Christians, take care of one another and the stranger in their midst. Many mountaineers believe that mental illness really has spiritual causes. Clarence Gray, better known as Catfish, Man of the Wood, is a herbalist who does some faith healing. He believes "that much of every illness is all in folks' minds and that guilt or anxiety from leading sinful lives contributes to many sicknesses" (Green 1978). Carole Hill, in her study of a folk medical belief system in the American South, observes that there is "the coexistence of two medical systems in American society (folk and orthodox). Obviously these two medical systems are not mutually exclusive" (Hill 1976, p. 14). She further recommends that there should be greater cooperation and mutual support between the two systems.

Appalachian folk medicine rests in part on religious beliefs. In the Bible, there are ninety-seven direct references to healing. Some of the more well-known biblical references in Appalachia concerning healing the sick are "See now that I, even I, am he, and there is no god beside me; I kill and I make alive; I wound and I heal" (Deuteronomy 32:39); "To one is given by the Spirit of the word of wisdom, to another the word of knowledge, to another faith, by the same Spirit the gifts of healing by the one Spirit" (I Corinthians 12:8-9); "There is a time and season for everything: A time to kill, a time to heal (Ecclesiastes 3:3); "Is any among you sick? Let him call for the elders of the church, and let them pray over him, anointing him with oil in the name of the Lord; and the prayer of faith will save the sick man, and the Lord will raise him up; and if he has committed sins, he will be forgiven. Therefore confess your sins to one another and pray for one another that you may be healed. The prayer of a righteous man has great power in its effects" (James 5:14-16). A number of Appalachian churches follow these verses literally in helping the sick.

Other churches follow rituals such as the flower service, foot washing, the kiss of peace, and the fellowship meetings, in which they confess sins, forgive one another, pray for one another, and use church discipline, if necessary. They believe that prayer is the weapon of God and thus can heal. They also believe Jesus, who said, "Your faith has healed you." They believe mental illness can be cured because, in Mark 5, Jesus cured the deranged man, one called Legion because he was possessed by so many demons. Moreover, the people accept the promise that runs through scriptures from Isaiah through Acts: if they should be converted, then they will be healed. Finally, the Bible gives the people the hope and promise that where medical science may fail, faith, prayer, and the ordinances of Jesus will not.

The attitudes held by traditional southern Appalachians make the services that mental health professionals offer difficult to accept. The counselor who is hostile or indifferent to the mountaineer's religion may feel the mountaineer's openness and trust turn into suspicion, hostility, and uncooperative behavior. Conversely, the mental health counselor who takes time to know the people, becomes personally concerned, and tries to maintain a nonjudgmental attitude toward established values will find clients open and cooperative.

Practical implications of the traditional southern Appalachian religion for mental health programs are numerous. The mental health professional is not only subject to the hostility or fear of the mountaineer but may also find that the mountaineer treats him or her as an equal. The mountaineers' Calvinist theology tends to have a leveling effect. Regardless of credentials, degrees, or titles, psychologists will fail if they do not relate to the family and its individual members on an informal and personal level. This means that one may have to counsel a family many times and win the family's trust before dealing with the given problem.

Therapists may also have to yield to the clients' belief in the authority of the Bible or personal experience over professional practice. For example, Ms. P., a social worker concerned with getting public assistance for the elderly, was very upset because she could not get a particular elderly couple to accept welfare, food stamps, or any kind of emergency assistance. She explained rationally, quoted the law, threatened, and finally broke down in tears imploring, "For God's sake, if you do not let me help you, you will starve to death. Please let me help you. I don't want you to die!" The man looked at his wife and said, "See, I told you she believed in God—she really does care for us." Then he turned to Ms. P. and said, "What do you want us to do?" Ms. P. was flabbergasted; the couple cooperated in every detail. Several months later, Ms. P. realized what had happened. She had become personal and even referred to God in her anger and frustration. The elderly couple interpreted this as sincere caring for them, especially when she asked God for help.

Ms. P. believes she has become more effective in her job, because she no longer deals with her clients as problems but as people. She now attempts to relate to her clients on a personal, religious, and family level. She says, "I now talk about their land, their family, their religion and, oh yes, the Bible." Ms. P. is Jewish, but she quotes the New Testament as well as the Old. She has found many scriptural passages that succinctly describe her job responsibilities. She particularly likes to quote Luke 4:18: "The Spirit of the Lord is upon me, because He has anointed me to preach good news to the poor. He has sent me to proclaim release to the captives and recovering of sight to the blind, to set at liberty those who are oppressed."

But the most effective passage she uses is Matthew 25:34-40: "Come, O Blessed of my Father, inherit the Kingdom prepared for you from the foundation of the world; for I was hungry and you gave me food, I was thirsty and you gave me drink, I was a stranger and you welcomed me, I was naked and you clothed me, I was sick and you visited me, I was in prison and you came to me. . . . Truly I say to you, as you did it to one of the least of these my brethren you did it to me."

Ms. P. has found that she must respect all persons, their culture and values, especially their religion. She believes that if she is to be effective in her work she must use the people's own frames of reference and sources of strength or security.

Accordingly, when mountain people say "we take care of our own," the counselor should accept that value. Through the development of a personal friendship or through scripture or the Calvinist theology, the worker may show that he or she is also one of "our" own and thus has a right "to take care of our own."

No professional should berate or ridicule another person's religion; on the other hand, one should not avoid religious topics, for as one mountaineer put it, "there ain't nothin' more personal than religion." Mountain people frequently discuss religion and even "bear witness" one to the other. A mature counselor must be a good listener and also be secure enough to state his or her own views without being dogmatic or afraid.

The mental health professional must realize that traditional mountain values are not simply old-fashioned but, from the mountaineers' perspective, are grounded in the Bible and thus are eternal. One must attempt to understand why mountain people act as they do. Once the source of their action has been identified (family, community, church, Bible, and so on), the counselor has also identified a source of strength through which to truly help clients. Specific problems continue to exist for regional agencies delivering services in the mountains:

1. Many people believe they are too poor to afford counseling;

2. Many people who could profit by treatment cannot stand up to the stigma of being labeled crazy;

3. People refuse to have family members placed in public institutions, especially mental institutions;

4. They do not want charity;

5. They will not trust agency personnel and thus they will not cooperate;

6. They prefer a local clinic over the county hospital or a state facility in the next county;

7. They refuse agency contact or cease cooperating when they do not see immediate results;

8. They cannot get excited about the agency's long-range impersonal objectives or goals;

9. They will not go to particular doctors or mental health professionals because, among other things, they may perceive counselors as atheists; they do not know the counselors personally; counselors are "from off"; and counselors are not considered friendly.

A common complaint in southern Appalachia concerning mental health services is illustrated by the following statement of Nancy Owens, a Christian Unity Baptist preacher:

Why, I went in there for help and they didn't say Hi! or nothin'. They stuck this paper under my nose, told me to fill it out (didn't even give me a pencil). When I'd done that, they begun asking me sech questions about my ma and pa and me. I got mad and left. I ain't no dog. I'm one of God's children. Why did they treat me that-a-way? That's what they always do. You go for help and instead you fill out forms or answer dumb questions. All they have to do is eyeball ya and say, "What's the trouble?" or "Can I help ya?" O' Lord, we would surely tell them if'n they had a mind to listen. [personal interview, August 12, 1979]

People in Appalachia find it difficult to understand why they have to go through so many steps before someone will finally deal directly with their problems. It is hard for them to see long-range goals or to understand the need for tests and government forms. In fact, many people are totally turned off by such procedures. Therapists should always try to establish rapport with a client before turning to required paperwork.

Counselors need local people to help them with the initial interview or contacts in order to help establish this rapport. David Looff (1971), a child psychiatrist, describes using this method very effectively. He has a local person working in each of his clinics and he makes his initial contacts through them. He uses local people he knows to make introductions for him when he is out in the community. In some cases, Looff uses local persons to assist in interviews, that is, getting descriptions of symptoms and possible treatments or solutions. Looff has found that the establishment of a trusting relationship is essential if one is to help traditional southern Appalachian people.[3]

If agency professionals are to help mountain people they must understand what their clients' words and actions are actually trying to convey to them; then, services may be offered in ways people can accept. Their place, their families, and their religion all are parts of a very intricate culture that must be respected and taken seriously. The professional must first come to know the person before being able to help the unique individual in southern Appalachia.

NOTES

1. Also see George L. Hicks (1976). Both of these authors emphasize the effect the family has upon the ethics of the people.

2. These passages are found in James 1:19, 2:1; Ephesians 4:26, 5:3; Colossians 3 and 4; I Thessalonians 3 and 4; II Timothy 2 and 3; and Titus 3.

3. Also see Looff (1977). This same theme runs through Robert Coles's book, volume 2 of *Children of crisis, Migrants, sharecroppers, mountaineers* (1971).

REFERENCES

Beaver, P.D. 1976. Symbols and social organization in an Appalachian mountain community. Ph.D. diss., Duke University, Durham.

Boles, J.B. 1972. *The Great Revival, 1787-1805*. Lexington: University Press of Kentucky.

Coles, R. 1971. *Children of crisis*, Vol. 2, *Migrants, sharecroppers, mountaineers*. Boston: Little, Brown.

Conn, C.W. 1977. *Like a mighty army*. Cleveland, Tenn.: Pathway Press.

Fetterman, J. 1967. *Stinking creek*. New York: E. P. Dutton.

Ford, T.R., ed. 1962. *The southern Appalachian region: A survey*. Lexington: University Press of Kentucky.

Green, E.C. 1978. A modern Appalachian folk healer. *Appalachian Journal* 6:12.

Hicks, G.L. 1976. *Appalachian valley*. New York: Holt, Rinehart and Winston.

Hill, C.E. 1976. A folk medical belief system in the American South: Some practical considerations. *Southern Medicine* 16:11-17.

Hooker, E.R. 1933. *Religion in the highlands*. New York: Home Missions Council.

Looff, D.H. 1971. *Appalachia's children*. Lexington: University Press of Kentucky.

Looff, D.H. 1977. Assisting Appalachian families. In *An Appalachia Symposium*, ed. J.W. Williamson, 102-12. Boone, N.C.: Appalachian State University Press.

Mauer, B.B. 1974. *Mountain heritage*. Morgantown, W.Va.: Morgantown Printing and Binding Co.

PART II

Sociocultural Systems and Mental Health Problems

4

Adaptive Socialization Values of Low-Income Appalachian Mothers

DAVID F. PETERS AND GARY W. PETERSON

The values that parents would like their children to adopt are significant influences in the parent-child relationship. An important focus of the research on this topic has been concerned with the links between aspects of the larger social structure (i.e., social class and culture) and parental socialization values (Ellis, Lee, and Peterson 1978; Gecas 1979; Inkeles 1969; Kohn 1977; Lee 1977; Pearlin 1971; Peterson, Lee, and Ellis 1982; Scheck and Emerick 1976; Wright and Wright 1976). That is, socioeconomic and subcultural groups differ in terms of the socialization values that parents convey to their offspring.

There are several reasons why the values that parents convey to their children are important considerations for mental health professionals working in Appalachia. First, parents are likely to translate these values into child-rearing practices that foster the social and personality characteristics they desire for their children (Kagan 1979; Martin 1975; Peterson and Rollins 1983; Rollins and Thomas 1979). For example, parents who value obedience in children might use higher levels of physical punishment, whereas parents who value the development of self-control might use higher levels of reasoning and negotiation with children. Second, some of these parental values and behaviors may be indicative of psychopathology (Walters and Walters 1980). Third, the values of many Appalachian parents may reflect cultural distinctions (Coles 1971; Ford 1962; Looff 1971; Polansky, Borgman, and De Saix 1972; Weller 1965) and be resistant to intervention procedures designed for the mainstream culture.

In the sociological literature, one of the principal investigators of parental socialization values has been Melvin Kohn (1959a, 1959b, 1963, 1969, 1977; Kohn and Schooler 1969), who has studied social class differences in the values that parents convey to their children during the socialization process. Using a sample from the Washington, D.C., area, Kohn (1969, 1977) focused on distinctions between the child-rearing values of middle- and working-class groups. His central idea was that the socioeconomic settings occupied by parents influence the socialization values they instill in their children. That is, parents tend to prepare their children ultimately to adapt to socioeconomic conditions similar to their own.

For example, those in middle-class occupations (e.g., white-collar supervisors, managers, and professionals) tend to emphasize abstract thinking, intellectual flexibility, and freedom from supervision. Experiences of this kind encourage middle-class parents to adopt socialization values emphasizing self-direction and internal standards of conduct. Conversely, those in blue-collar and low-income occupations (e.g., factory workers, operators, laborers) usually require the manipulation of physical objects, greater standardization of tasks, less intellectual flexibility, and closer supervision. As a result of these and other conditions of life, blue-collar parents tend to value obedience, conformity, and neatness in their children. Values such as these are probably adaptive in light of the harsh conditions confronting parents and children from lower socioeconomic backgrounds (Gecas 1979; Peterson and Rollins 1983).

Although large samples with diverse characteristics have been used to study parents' socialization values (Gecas and Nye 1974; Scheck and Emerick 1976; Wright and Wright 1976), this topic has not been a subject of concern in studies of Appalachian parents. The major purpose of this study, therefore, was to compare the socialization values of mothers from low-income families in rural Appalachia with the socialization values of urban middle- and working-class mothers from Kohn's (1969, 1977) Washington, D.C., sample.

In addition to Kohn's work on social class and maternal values, it is also important to consider the existing literature on the child-rearing processes within low-income Appalachian families. Child-rearing values in Appalachia, for example, retain an adult-centered focus, in which children are expected to obey their parents and conform to the expectations of adults (Looff 1971; Weller 1965). Appalachian youth from low-income families are exposed to unusually strong familistic orientations and parental practices that encourage family closeness and dependency on parents (Ford 1962; Heller and Quesada 1977; Looff 1971; Photiadis 1980). Such descriptions point out that low-income Appalachian parents, like Kohn's sample of urban blue-collar workers, may emphasize conformity and obedience in their parenting. Thus, in keeping with Kohn's (1969, 1977) socioeconomic distinctions, low-income white mothers from rural Appalachia would be expected to differ from urban middle-class mothers in the priorities they assign to several child-rearing values, primarily in assigning higher priority to the values of obedience, conformity to others, and neatness in children. Low-income Appalachian mothers also would be expected to give lower priority to such child-rearing values as self-direction, internal dynamics, happiness, and curiosity than urban middle-class mothers.

The possibility also existed, however, that the value priorities of low-income mothers from Appalachia would differ in degree of intensity from Kohn's (1969, 1977) sample of mothers from urban blue-collar backgrounds. Although the mothers in Kohn's Washington, D.C., study were from families in which the fathers held stable, blue-collar occupations (such as factory workers, mill operators, construction workers, and clerical personnel) the sample for the present study was composed of Appalachian mothers from a category of disadvantaged families whose economic plight has been well documented (Caudill 1962, 1976; Coles 1971; Looff 1971; Polansky et al. 1972; Weller 1965). Consistent with a proposal by Gecas (1979), therefore, economically deprived mothers would be expected to have child-rearing values that were more extreme versions of blue-collar values. Consequently, the child-rearing values of low-income Appalachian mothers surveyed in this investigation were expected to demonstrate even greater orientation toward obedience and conformity than those of the urban blue-collar mothers interviewed by Kohn. Low-income Appalachian mothers also were expected to give lower priority to socialization values concerned with self-direction and internal dynamics than urban blue-collar mothers.

SAMPLE AND METHOD

Data for this study were acquired as part of the Southern Occupational Goals Study, an investigation of fifth- and sixth-grade students and their mothers from low-income backgrounds. A sample of 1202 low-income black mothers (623) and white mothers (579) was acquired as part of a research project conducted in six states in the southeastern region of the United States (Kentucky, Mississippi, North Carolina, South Carolina, Tennessee, and Virginia).

A subsample from the larger project was used for the present study, consisting of 579 low-income white mothers (287 having a male and

292 a female child) from rural, Appalachian counties (containing towns of 2500 or fewer residents) in Kentucky, North Carolina, and Tennessee. Both the mothers and their husbands were employed in the lower five levels of the United States Census Bureau's occupational classification. More specifically, they were employed as craftsmen, operatives in factories, laborers, clerical workers, service workers, and agriculture workers. All of the women included in the sample were the mothers of fifth- and sixth-grade children (mean age, 11.2 years), who attended schools that were selected for the project (see Southern Regional Research Project S-63, 1974). The average educational attainment of these low-income women was 8.6 years of formal schooling.

A nonprobability sampling design was used for the larger project. The first phase involved the selection of twenty urban and rural schools from economically depressed areas within the six participating states. Selected schools were located in counties characterized by high levels of unemployment, poverty, and school drop-outs. In addition, schools considered in this study were selected based on a stratification of rural areas containing towns of 2500 or fewer residents. To meet sampling quotas within each state, the number of schools actually chosen corresponded to the selection of approximately one out of three that met the stratification criteria for the project. Given a balance of stratified school choices with clusters of students selected within schools, it is suggested that sampling error estimation based on a simple random sampling model was a realistic approximation (see Howell and Frese 1981; Proctor 1974). Significance tests based on this assumption, however, should be treated with caution.

All fifth- and sixth-grade students who attended the selected schools on the day of the survey were administered the Otis-Lennon Mental Ability Test (Otis and Lennon 1967, 1969) as a means of screening out children who were unable to respond effectively to the questionnaire. Because the objectives of this project concerned low-income samples, children and parents of higher socioeconomic status were excluded from the sample, based on the parents' occupational status and educational attainment. The final 1202 mother-child pairs represented 58% of all the children who were available initially in the fifth- and sixth-grade classrooms of the selected schools. In the present study, data acquired from the sample of rural low-income Appalachian mothers (from towns of 2500 residents or less) were compared with working- and middle-class samples of mothers that Kohn (1969, 1977) interviewed in Washington, D.C. Kohn characterized the mothers of this sample as having husbands whose occupational categories included operatives, laborers, craftsmen, and foremen.

Children who participated in the study responded to a questionnaire that was read aloud to them in school classrooms, while mothers were interviewed in their homes by trained investigators. Only the responses of mothers concerning their socialization values were pertinent to the present study. The method used to assess these values corresponded closely with Kohn's (1969, 1977) procedures and consisted of a question requesting that mothers choose three characteristics (from 16 possibilities) that they valued in their children. During the structured interview, the mothers were handed a card and told: "This card has sixteen statements. I am going to read all of them first and then you tell me the three that you think are the most important for a boy (girl) the age of (the child's name)." Socialization values that the mothers had the option to select were is happy, is considerate of others, has self-control, tries hard to succeed, is dependable, is interested in why and how things work, is honest, is a good student, obeys parents well, is clean and neat, gets along well with others, has good manners, is affectionate, is liked by adults, is able to defend self, and acts in a serious way. Items which Kohn identified as representing a conformity-obedience orientation were: obeys parents well, is clean and neat, has good manners, and is a good student.[1] Responses identified as representing self-direction and internalization were: is happy, is considerate of others, has self-control, is dependable, and is interested in how and why things work.

Some of the value items in Kohn's Washington, D.C., study were altered for clarity in accordance with later research by Kohn on a national sample. Instead of the item "the child is popular with other children," the phrase "gets along well with other children" was employed. Second, the "ambitious" item was replaced by the response "tries hard to succeed." Third, the response "curious" was changed to "is interested in why and how things happen." Finally, the item "is able to play by himself/herself" was not included in the project questionnaire, consistent with Kohn's decision to drop this item in later research.

Significance tests for the differences between two proportions were used to examine whether systematic differences existed in maternal values between each of the two samples of low-income mothers and the samples of urban middle- and working-class mothers from Kohn's (1969, 1977) research. Separate comparisons were made between the value selections of mothers of girls and mothers of boys.

Table 4.1 Socialization Value Choices by Urban Middle-Class Mothers and Rural Low-Income Appalachian Mothers

	Mother of Boys			Mother of Girls		
Socialization Value	Appalachian Low-Income %		Urban (Kohn's) Middle-Class %	Appalachian Low-Income %		Urban (Kohn's) Middle-Class %
Obedience-Conformity						
Obeys parents well	44	**	18	44	**	23
Gets along well with others (popular)	45	**	13	44	**	17
Is clean and neat	10		07	25	*	15
Has good manners	14		16	25		23
Is a good student	21		17	25	**	13
Self-Direction/Internalization						
Is happy	20	**	44	18	**	48
Is considerate of others	10	**	40	14	**	38
Has self-control	10	**	24	07	*	20
Is dependable	18	*	27	17		20
Is interested in why and how things happen (curious)	13		20	13		15
Other						
Tries hard to succeed	28	**	09	22	**	06
Is honest	54		44	47		44
N	287		90	292		84

Note: Low proportions and no significant differences were found for the items "able to defend self," "affectionate," "liked by adults," "acts in a serious way."
*p < .05.
**p < .01.

RESULTS

Table 4.1 shows the proportions of mothers assessed for this study from low-income Appalachian backgrounds and urban middle-class mothers from Kohn's (1969, 1977) research who selected a particular child characteristic (or socialization value) as one of their three choices. Comparisons are shown separately for mothers of boys and mothers of girls.

As expected, the low-income Appalachian mothers demonstrate greater obedience-conformity orientation than middle-class mothers. Specifically, five of six comparisons involving the "obeys parents well," "gets along well with others," and "is clean and neat" are consistent with this pattern. Further evidence of a conformity orientation is the greater choice of the "is a good student" value by low-income mothers of girls as compared to urban middle-class mothers.

Also consistent with prediction are the tendencies for Appalachian mothers to select values that measure self-direction and internal values less frequently than urban mothers. In seven of eight comparisons, the rural Appalachian mothers choose the "is happy," "is considerate of others," "has self-control," and "is dependable" values less frequently than urban middle-class mothers.

The three value items most frequently selected by Appalachian mothers of boys and girls are "is honest," "obeys parents well," and "gets along well with others." An unexpected finding is that low-income Appalachian mothers of boys and girls select the "tries hard to succeed" values in greater proportions than middle-income mothers.

Table 4.2 displays the value choices of low-income Appalachian mothers as compared to the choices of urban working-class mothers. As expected, low-income Appalachian mothers demonstrate a conformity-obedience orientation in choosing the values "obeys parents well," "gets along well with others," and "is a good student" more frequently than urban working-class mothers in four of six possible comparisons. Other choices by Appalachian mothers demonstrate the expected differences in regard to internal dynamics and self-direction. Specifically, in four of six comparisons, low-income Appalachian mothers choose the "is happy," "is considerate of others," and "is dependable" values less frequently than working-class mothers. Table 4.2 also displays the unexpected finding that Appalachian mothers of girls and boys select the "tries hard to succeed" value more often than urban blue-collar mothers.

Table 4.2. Socialization Value Choices by Urban Working-Class Mothers and Rural Low-Income Appalachian Mothers

	Mother of Boys			Mother of Girls		
Socialization Value	Appalachian Low-Income %		Urban (Kohn's) Working-Class %	Appalachian Low-Income %		Urban (Kohn's) Working-Class %
Obedience-Conformity						
Obeys parents well	44		37	44	*	30
Gets along well with others (popular)	45	**	15	44	**	20
Is clean and neat	10		13	25		28
Has good manners	14		17	25	*	32
Is a good student	21		23	25		11
Self Direction/Internalization						
Is happy	20		27	18	**	45
Is considerate of others	10	**	30	14	*	24
Has self-control	10	*	14	07		13
Is dependable	18		27	17		14
Is interested in why and how things happen (curious)	13		06	13		07
Other						
Tries hard to succeed	28	*	18	22	**	08
Is honest	54		57	47		48
N	287		90	292		84

Note: Low proportions and no significant differences were found for the items "able to defend self," "affectionate," "liked by adults," "acts in a serious way."
*p < .05.
**p < .01.

DISCUSSION

In general, the results of this study are consistent with both the present research expectations and earlier investigations on parental socialization values (Gecas and Nye 1974; Kohn 1969, 1977). That is, these findings provide some evidence linking socioeconomic conditions to parental socialization values that may be adaptive within the context of rural Appalachia. To the extent that parents succeed in fostering these valued outcomes in children, they are likely to encourage cross-generational similarity in occupational attainment, conditions of life, and socialization attitudes.

The data in Tables 4.1 and 4.2 reveal consistent patterns in the values chosen by the sample of mothers. Although not all of the comparisons are significant, those that reached significant levels are in the expected direction. Appalachian mothers from low-income areas are more likely to select conformity-obedience values and less likely to select values representing self-direction and internalization than urban middle-class mothers. Low-income Appalachian mothers, furthermore, respond as expected by choosing conformity-obedience values more frequently and self-control, internalization values less frequently than urban blue-collar mothers (Gecas 1979). In other words, although differing in magnitude, the general pattern of the Appalachian mothers' value choices (i.e., higher obedience-conformity values and lower self-direction, internalization values) is similar to value choices made by other mothers from lower socioeconomic levels located elsewhere in the United States. Previous accounts of certain "unique" aspects of Appalachian life (Looff 1971, Polansky et al. 1972; Weller 1965), consequently, may actually be a product of socioeconomic rather than subcultural circumstances. For example, the conformity and obedience orientations of Appalachian parents (that are supposed to be a part of Appalachian familistic orientations) may actually be a product of social class rather than subcultural conditions (c.f., Hennon and Photiadis 1979; Looff 1971; Weller 1965). Both low-income parents in general and families from Appalachia have been described as being concerned especially with the actions and outcomes of their offspring. Children are socialized by, watched over by, and are clearly subordinate to parents and extended kin. Few decisions are made by the young without the knowledge and participation of parents and other family members (Polansky et al. 1972; Schwarzweller, Brown, and Mangalam 1971).

Other value selections by Appalachian mothers that differ from

Kohn's results, on the other hand, may be explained by regional uniqueness rather than socioeconomic circumstances. For example, descriptions of low-income Appalachian family members as being fatalistic seem consistent with the tendency for them to select the values "has self-control" and "is happy" less frequently (Ford 1962; Polansky et al. 1972; Weller 1965). Instead of viewing this orientation as problematic (Lesser 1970), however, fatalism is conceptualized here as a realistic response to the special conditions faced by low-income Appalachian families. As suggested by Lewis and Knipe (1978), fatalism or a feeling of powerlessness is an adjustive response to outside interests who control the institutions and economy of Appalachia. Outside control of this kind creates the conditions for high levels of poverty, political domination by outside interests, and exploitation. Fatalism is one means that Appalachians may use to protect their way of life from new economic models and the concomitant intrusion of an alien culture from outside their region.

Descriptions of Appalachians as being person-oriented also seem consistent with the propensity of these mothers to select the "gets along well with others" value quite frequently (Ford 1962; Weller 1965). That is, a value selection of this kind may reflect the ethic of neutrality or the emphasis on harmony reported to exist in the social relationships of rural Appalachians. According to this conception, expectations for social interaction with others include proscriptions against raising controversies, initiating conflict, becoming aggressive, or exercising authority over others (Hicks 1976).

The unexpected finding that Appalachian mothers frequently select the "tries hard to succeed" value may reflect an interpretation Kohn offers in his research. In this case, low-income Appalachian mothers may place special emphasis on this value because they recognize that "success" is an especially difficult attainment in the rural South, an area characterized by high levels of poverty and few employment opportunities (Chadwick and Bahr 1978; Ford 1978). Consistent with Kohn's (1977) idea, therefore, low-income mothers may give special priority to the "tries hard to succeed" value because they view the likelihood of their children's success as being especially problematic. Disadvantaged mothers from Appalachia apparently want to capitalize as much as possible on their children's opportunity for success—however slim it may be—by placing strong emphasis on this value.

Corresponding with this interpretation are findings that low-income parents often have high aspirations for their children, despite the harsh realities they face (Thomas and Falk 1978). An alternative explanation might be that a success orientation of this kind is more characteristic of parents living in rural than in urban environments. Miller and Swanson (1958), for example, propose that parents from rural environments are more likely to be influenced by the individualistic and entrepreneurial orientations that are more common in agricultural than urban settings.

Although the present results provide substantial evidence indicating that socialization values may be linked to the life circumstances of low-income families, the selection of the "tries hard to succeed" value also raises some doubts about the efficacy of culture of poverty or similar theories that attribute parental child-rearing values to class determinism. That is, the selection of this "success" value by Appalachian mothers from rural areas is more reflective of a middle-class orientation than values that are supposed to be typical of either working-class or culture-of-poverty orientations. This instead may be an example of a "dual orientation," in which low-income mothers acknowledge the need for surface conformity by their children as an adaptive mechanism within the immediate socioeconomic context while maintaining a desire for their children to rise above their current circumstances. Such a dual orientation by parents involves recognition of both the value of success in the larger society and the structural limitations that their own children are likely to face in the future. That is, the desire for success remains evident among these mothers despite such obstacles as inadequate schools, few occupational opportunities, and limited economic resources (Durant and Knowlton 1978; Hennon and Photiadis 1979). Adopting this dual orientation, however, may form the basis for later psychological difficulties in some Appalachian children. The combination of values related to obedience, conformity, and a desire to succeed may lead to adult conflicts, when the motivation to succeed is incompatable with the likely attainment of manual level jobs.

Results of this kind about maternal values have important implications for mental health professionals who work with Appalachian families. That is, surveys have consistently found that high levels of psychological disorders are prevalent among low-income Appalachians and other disadvantaged groups (Dohrenwend and Dohrenwend 1969, 1974; Polansky et al. 1972). Characteristic life-style and value systems of low-income Appalachians, such as cohesive family ties and social and geographic isoation, insulate members of Appalachian families from community agencies and mental health professionals. The inexpressive qualities of Appalachian mothers,

furthermore, may contribute to difficulties in types of therapy requiring effective communication skills on the part of clients (Haley
1976; Korchin 1980; Looff 1971; Polansky et al. 1972).

In other words, mental health professionals will be more successful
if the values and life-styles of Appalachian clients are reflected in the
kinds of interventions used. For example, directive techniques may
be successful because they require therapists to assume a supervisory
role within the therapeutic relationship and to specify that clients
conform to their expectations. Similar to other low-income groups,
Appalachian family members may respond more favorably to interventions of this kind rather than nondirective techniques (Korchin
1980). That is, clinicians may be less successful when they focus exclusively on the phenomenological world of Appalachian clients in
the manner of traditional psychotherapies. Instead, the effectiveness
of therapy might be enhanced if traditional approaches are combined
with advice giving, vocational guidance, and financial counseling as
a means of assisting clients with some of the harsh realities of their
low-income circumstances. Interventions with low-income Appalachian families, furthermore, might be more successful when carried
out in the home. By developing programs that are implemented
within the familiar context of the family, many of the difficulties associated with social and geographic isolation may be surmounted.

Another issue raised by the present findings concerns the relevance
of current parent education programs to low-income families from
Appalachia. Because middle-class child-rearing values form the bases
of many parent education programs (Harman and Brim 1980), they
frequently emphasize the importance of encouraging self-direction,
achievement, and other middle-class values. The low-income Appalachian mothers studied here, in contrast, indicate a consistent preference for conformity-obedience orientations combined with an
emphasis on success. To address this dual orientation, parent edu-
cators who work with Appalachian parents might design parenting
programs that recognize the importance of conformity to parents,
while encouraging the value of achievement in settings beyond the
family. Intervention programs of this kind will be compatible both
with the values of Appalachian family life and the desire for attainment in the larger culture.

Additional implications for mental health research and training programs can be derived from the finding that maternal socialization
values were focused on preparing offspring for adjustments to both
the Appalachian and mainstream cultures. Conventional research in

psychology, for example, has concentrated on developing panhuman principles of behavior (Kagan 1979; Kessen 1979), but little knowledge exists regarding the important distinctions in personality organization, differential manifestations of pathology, and selective responsivity to different interventions by members of various subcultural groups (Korchin 1980). Moreover, very few clinical training programs deal specifically with issues pertaining to the values of minority and other subcultural groups (Bernard and Padilla 1982).

In order to provide effective mental health care, greater emphasis in training and research should be placed on the sociocultural influences that affect the values and behavior of low-income Appalachian parents and children. Training programs for mental health professionals in Appalachia, for example, might adopt a multicultural approach combining both the special concerns of rural Appalachia and the therapeutic procedures used with American families in the larger culture. Clinicians thus may design intervention strategies that enable Appalachian families to deal more effectively with the harsh realities of low-income rural life and also establish constructive links with mainstream America. Interventions of this kind capitalize on the desires of low-income Appalachian parents to socialize their children for living both within the contexts of rural Appalachia and the larger culture.

NOTES

Funding for this research was provided by the Agricultural Experiment Station, The University of Tennessee, Knoxville, Projects S-63, S-126, and S-171.

1. In a comparative study of Italian and American parents, Kohn (1969, 1977) concluded that the "good student" value reflected a "conformity" orientation toward school requirements.

REFERENCES

Bernard, M.E., and M.E. Padilla. 1982. Status of minority curricula and training in clinical psychology. *American Psychologist* 37(7):780-87.
Caudill, H.M. 1962. *Night comes to the Cumberlands*. Boston: Little, Brown.
Caudill, H.M. 1976. *The watches of the night*. Boston: Little, Brown.
Chadwick, B.A., and H.M. Bahr. 1978. Rural poverty. In *Rural U.S.A.: Persistence and change*, ed. T.R. Ford. Ames: Iowa State University Press.
Coles, R.W 1971. *Children of crisis*, vol. 2. *Migrants, share croppers, mountaineers*. Boston: Little, Brown.
Dohrenwend, B.P., and B.S. Dohrenwend. 1969. *Social status and psychological disorder*. New York: Wiley.

Dohrenwend, B.P., and B.S. Dohrenwend. 1974. Social and cultural influences on psychopathology. *Annual Review of Psychology* 25:417-52.

Durant, T.J., and C.S. Knowlton. 1978. Rural ethnic minorities: Adaptive responses to inequality. In *Rural U.S.A.: Persistence and change*, ed. T.R. Ford. Ames: Iowa State University Press.

Ellis, G.J., G.R. Lee, and L.R. Peterson. 1978. Supervision and conformity: A cross-cultural analysis of parental socialization values. *American Journal of Sociology* 84:386-403.

Ford, T.R., ed. 1962. *The southern Appalachian region: A survey.* Lexington: University Press of Kentucky.

Ford, T.R., ed. 1978. *Rural U.S.A.: Persistence and change.* Ames: Iowa State University Press.

Gecas, V. 1979. The influence of social class on socialization. In *Contemporary theories about the family* vol. 2, eds. W.R. Burr, R. Hill, F.I. Nye, and I.L. Reiss. New York: Free Press.

Gecas, V., and F.I. Nye. 1974. Sex and class differences in parent-child interaction: A test of Kohn's hypothesis. *Journal of Marriage and the Family* 36:742-49.

Haley, J. 1976. *Problem-solving therapy.* San Francisco: Jossey-Bass.

Harman, D., and O.G. Brim. 1980. *Learning to be parents: Principles, programs, and methods.* Beverly Hills, Calif.: Sage Publications.

Heller, P.L., and G.M. Quesada. 1977. Rural familism: An interregional analysis. *Rural Sociology* 42:220-40.

Hennon, C.B., and J. Photiadis. 1979. The rural Appalachian low-income male: Changing role in a changing family. *Family Coordinator* 28:608-15.

Hicks, G. 1976. *Appalachian valley.* New York: Holt, Rinehart and Winston.

Howell, F.M., and W. Frese. 1981. Educational plans as motivation or attitude: Some additional evidence. *Social Psychology Quarterly* 44:218-36.

Inkeles, A. 1969. Social structure and socialization. In *Handbook of socialization theory and research*, ed. D.A. Goslin. Chicago: Rand McNally.

Kagan, J. 1979. Family experience and the child's development. *American Psychologist* 34(10):886-91.

Kessen, W. 1979. The American child and other cultural inventions. *American Psychologist* 34(10):815-20.

Kohn, M. 1959a. Socialization, class and parental values. *American Journal of Sociology* 64:337-51.

Kohn, M. 1959b. Social class and the experience of parental authority. *American Sociological Review* 24:352-66.

Kohn, M. 1963. Social class and parent-child relationships: An interpretation. *American Journal of Sociology* 68: 470-80.

Kohn, M. 1969. *Class and conformity: A study in values.* Homewood, Ill.: Dorsey Press.

Kohn, M. 1977. *Class and conformity: A study in values.* 2nd ed. Chicago: University of Chicago Press.

Kohn, M., and C. Schooler. 1969. Class, occupation and orientation. *American Sociological Review* 34:659-78.

Korchin, S.J. 1980. Clinical psychology and minority problems. *American Psychologist* 35(3):262-69.

Lee, G.R. 1977. *Family structure and interaction: A comparative analysis.* Philadelphia: J.B. Lippincott.

Lesser, G. 1970. Culture: Toward tomorrow's people. *People's Appalachia* 1(1):10-20.

Lewis, H.M., and E.E. Knipe. 1978. The colonialism model: The Appalachian case. In *Colonialism in modern America: The Appalachian case*, eds. H.M. Lewis, L. Johnson and D. Askins. Boone, N.C.: Appalachian Consortium Press.

Looff, D.H. 1971. *Appalachia's children: The challenge of mental health*. Lexington: University Press of Kentucky.

Martin, B. 1975. Parent-child relations. In *Review of child development research*, ed. R.D. Horowitz. Chicago: University of Chicago Press.

Miller, D.R., and G.E. Swanson. 1958. *The changing American parent*. New York: Wiley.

Otis, A., and R. Lennon. 1967. *Otis-Lennon mental ability test*. New York: Harcourt, Brace and World.

Otis, A., and R. Lennon. 1969. *Otis-Lennon technical handbook*. New York: Harcourt, Brace and World.

Pearlin, L. 1971. *Class context and family relationships: A cross-national study*. Boston: Little, Brown.

Peterson, G.W., and B.C. Rollins. 1983. Parent-child socialization and symbolic interaction. In *Handbook of marriage and the family*, eds. M.B. Sussman and S.K. Steinmetz. New York: Plenum Press.

Peterson, L.R., G.R. Lee, and G.J. Ellis. 1982. Social structure, socialization values and disciplinary techniques: A cross-cultural analysis. *Journal of Marriage and the Family* 44:131-42.

Photiadis, J.D. 1980. *The changing rural Appalachian and low-income family: Implications for community development*, West Virginia University Bulletin, Series 80, No. 7-9. Morgantown: Office of Research and Development, West Virginia University.

Polansky, N.A., R.D. Borgman, and C. De Saix. 1972. *Roots of futility*. San Francisco: Jossey-Bass.

Proctor, C. 1974. Methodology for the baseline study. In *Influences on the occupational goals of young people in three southern subcultures*, Southern Regional Research Project S-63. Greensboro, N.C.: Agriculture Experiment Station.

Rollins, B.C., and D.L. Thomas. 1979. Parental support, power, and control techniques in the socialization of children. In *Contemporary theories about the family: Research based theories*, vol. 1, eds. W.R. Burr, R. Hill, F.I. Nye, and I.L. Reiss. New York: Free Press.

Scheck, D.C., and R. Emerick. 1976. The young male adolescent's perception of early childrearing behavior: The differential effects of socioeconomic status and family size. *Sociometry* 39:39-52.

Schwarzweller, H.K., J.S. Brown, and J.J. Mangalam. 1971. *Mountain families in transition*. University Park: Pennsylvania State University Press.

Southern Regional Research Project S-63. 1974. *Influences on the occupational goals of young people in three southern subcultures*. Knoxville, Tenn.: Agriculture Experiment Station.

Thomas, J.K., and W.W. Falk. 1978. Career attitudes and achievements. In *Education and work in rural America: The social context of early career decisions and achievement*, eds. A.G. Cosby and I. Charney. Houston: Stafford-Lowdon.

Walters, J., and L.H. Walters. 1980. Parent-child relationships: A review, 1970-1979. *Journal of Marriage and the Family* 42:807-22.

Weller, J. 1965. *Yesterday's people*. Lexington: University Press of Kentucky.

Wright, J.D., and S.R. Wright. 1976. Social class and parental values for children: A partial replication and extension of Kohn's thesis. *American Sociological Review* 41:527-37.

5

Gender, Class and Self-Image

JUDITH IVY FIENE

Little systematic attention has been given to the importance of gender in determining the individual life course in Appalachia (Tickamyer and Tickamyer 1987; Walls and Billings 1977). Little data is available on female-headed households and there is a paucity of statistical data regarding Appalachian women in general (Weeks 1980). Analyses of social structure in Appalachian communities frequently define women's lives solely in relation to their position or role functions within the traditional family group (Photiadis 1986; Stephenson 1968; Schwarzweller, Brown, and Mangalam 1971).

Low-status Appalachian women, in particular, have been typically represented by stereotypical images not only in the media but, at times, in the professional literature of the past fifty years. Images of this type are still prevalent in some programs serving the rural poor and can structure the quality of institutional interactions with the women themselves. Such images fail to communicate the diversity of interests, skills, and abilities among women in this segment of the society. Frequently overlooked is the flexibility women display in response to their stressful environment and the strength that some have gained through adversity.

This chapter examines the impact of both gender and social status on the mental health of low-status rural Appalachian women. It will review the images of low-status women presented in contemporary Appalachian studies literature and the sources of some common stereotypes. Descriptions of low-status women derived from the following four sources will be addressed: (1) sociological and anthropological studies that map social stratification and social structure in rural Appalachian communities, (2) studies of the psychological characteristics of Appalachian women and their families, (3) social science studies concerned with the impact of the political and economic dynamics of the region on its people, and (4) accounts of the lives of individual women contained in oral histories or biographies.

Whatever the source, descriptions of a group of people, such as low-status women, can become static, frozen in their spot in time. Considerable intellectual energy is then expended in attempting to determine how and why the women have developed as they have. Because it is not possible to see the people they will become, it is easy to overlook the fact that they may change, mature, learn from experience. Their own perspective on who they have become and how they define themselves, will be addressed using an analysis of the self-descriptions of some low-status women as contained in their life stories. The chapter will conclude with an assessment of the implications of these varied perspectives for the mental health of low-status women.

SOCIAL STATUS IN RURAL COMMUNITIES

Discussions of women in the majority of ethnography and sociological studies focused on Appalachia are embedded in analyses and descriptions of the family. Recognizing the prevalence of familism in the region (Heller and Quesada 1977), these studies concentrate their attention on either the kinship network or the generative family: parents and minor children. Low-status women may be perceived in their rural communities in terms of the, often derogatory, labels placed on their kinship group or they may be categorized as members of families clinging to traditional mountain values.

Studies in isolated mountain communities with a high degree of kinship have found that the ideal of egalitarianism, merging with the need for cooperation, minimizes the stratification process while blunting intragroup aggression (Beaver 1976, 1986; Hicks 1976). Even these closely knit communities, however, are socially stratified, and women or men who are deemed to be lazy, unwilling to work, or prone to dependency on social agencies are at the bottom of the group socially and economically and are labeled worthless by the larger community (Beaver 1976). In such communities, where close scrutiny of behavior is inevitable due to the small size of the group, problematic behavior is tied to deviations from the group work ethic.

Closely associated with this perspective is another form of labeling applied to women identified as members of stigmatized families with a multigenerational history of "sorry" behavior. Female "sorry" behavior has been said to include promiscuity, social dependency, alcoholism, and inadequate mothering (Cavender 1981; Hicks 1976). The existence of expectations based on community experience with earlier generations of an individual's family creates the possibility of qualitative differences in interactions with these individuals across their life span: in school, church, etc. Labeling by family association can lead to the maintenance of the social status quo, influence the development of self-identity in low-status youth, and probably controls the nature of the resources made available to individuals in this group.

Other ethnographic studies in Appalachia have reported a clearer stratification system with some variation of high, middle- and low-strata (Keefe, Reck, and Reck 1985; Schwarzweller et al. 1971; Stephenson 1968). A common assumption has been that the critical demarcation between social strata is determined by each group's level of adaptation to the norms and life styles of the urban middle class. Low-status groups are seen as least assimilated to the new norms and women in this category are said to be more bound by traditional sex-role mores (Kaplan 1971; Photiadis 1970). Traditional female role behavior, restrictions in the choice of role models, and limited employment opportunities are all seen as factors affecting the occupational aspirations of women (Photiadis 1986).

A composite picture of the low-status woman, drawn from the types of studies just discussed, portrays a socially isolated woman whose role choices are limited to those of homemaker and mother except in the face of serious economic necessity. She is seldom self-assertive and chooses to avoid problematic situations. She may be content with her lot in life or fatalistic about God's will. There is a high probability that she is dependent, at some time, on community social services and has more children than the national average. At various times in her life, she may exhibit symptoms related to chronic stress and depression. She may become the victim of family violence and yet be unable to act decisively for herself. Her inexperience in the larger social world makes it difficult for her to deal with impersonal representatives of assisting agencies.

The multiple sources of stress in rural poverty families has been delineated by Fitchen (1981). Parents are portrayed as struggling through economic losses and unemployment, overcrowded and in-adequate housing, acute disruptions in the marital relationship, and the myriad problems presented by illness to maintain the family unit at all costs. A similar scene was observed in southern Appalachia by Coles (1971). When the family unit remains the focus of attention, however, the specific position of women is often obscured. Given the socialization of American women as the guardians of the family's emotional welfare, women in poor families would seem to occupy a dangerously stressful position in our social world.

PSYCHOLOGICAL PERSPECTIVES

Specific personality traits have been associated with low-status women. Ball (1968) and Photiadis (n.d.) suggested that a lack of integration into mainstream cultural norms and perceptions of social and economic deprivation have created specific personality attributes and values in low-status individuals. In this model low-status women are said to evidence resignation, fatalism, apathy, and frustration while displaying social dependency, a present orientation with the seeking of immediate gratification, alcoholism, fecundity, and low levels of education. Attributions of this type are a mixture of concepts drawn from descriptions of regional personality characteristics thought to constitute an Appalachian subculture (Weller 1965), and studies of the characteristics of poverty families (Parenstedt 1965), typical of research using the culture of poverty model. This model has been criticized extensively and its deleterious applications to the Appalachian population have been reviewed by writers including Fisher (1977) and Walls and Billings (1977).

Two prominent studies, conducted in the early 1970s, touch on the socialization process in low-income or low-status rural Appalachian families. Although these studies are concerned with special populations, families with psychologically disturbed children (Looff 1971), and neglectful mothers (Polansky, Borgman, and De Saix 1972), their conclusions have influenced present-day images of low-status Appalachian women.

Looff (1971), a psychiatrist, concluded that the most common mental health problems in rural Appalachia are school-phobia, overly dependent personality disorders, conversion reactions and hysterical personality disorders, and elective mutism. Women, viewed in their maternal role, are described as so nurturing, warm, and indulgent (a personality strength) that many of them end up being overprotective, particularly of male children (potentially pathogenic). Other negative results of this strong orientation to feelings are said to be a lack of control of aggressive impulses and reduced verbal communication.

In addressing the special problems of the very poor, Looff warns against generalizations regarding poverty populations, pointing to the diversity of experience in differing environments. He also recognizes the role of insufficient economic opportunities and resources in creating stresses that are interactive with individual personality configurations.

Polansky et al. (1972) paint a negative picture of an intergenerational cycle of poverty and futility stemming from pervasive inadequacies in maternal personality, resulting in serious child neglect. Subscribing to subcultural theory, the authors identify four cultural themes said to be both regressive and distinctive of Appalachian culture. These are infantilization of males; separation anxiety, conformity, and fusion fantasies; inexpressiveness; and fatalism. Polansky et al.'s study is significant both because it labels Appalachian mothers and traditional family styles as pathogenic and also because the paucity of subsequent research has left these conclusions unchallenged in psychological literature. As such, it has contributed to the stereotype of low-status Appalachian women.

ECONOMIC DYNAMICS

The impact of economic exploitation and cultural imperialism on the welfare of Appalachian communities and families has been extensively described (Gaventa 1980; Lewis and Knipe 1978). These observers locate the economic problems of the Appalachian region in the usurping of the area's resources by outside moneyed interests and depict the region's women and men as powerless to control the nature or profits of their labor (Lewis and Knipe 1978).

Strategies for coping with their environment may place low-status women in conflict with the community representatives commissioned to assist them. The source of this conflict is seen to result from the historical incompatibility between traditional mountain women and their values (simplicity, cooperation, egalitarianism, and familism) and the values of the newcomers to the region at the end of the nineteenth century (hard work, education, cleanliness, and competitiveness). The unsophisticated mountain woman encountered a powerful new role model in the missionaries, teachers, and nurses who came to the area. What ensued, unfortunately, has been a continual denigration of the indigenous culture leaving the natives on the defensive.

From this perspective, local cultural patterns, such as passive behavior and fatalistic attitudes, are functional coping mechanisms developed in the face of external threats to existence and serve to preserve the family unit as a refuge for individuals powerless to change a hostile environment (Lewis, Kobak, and Johnson 1978). Families become resistent to change and encourage child behaviors that increase family harmony while rejecting outside social institutions. For example, maternal overprotection, which is defined as problematic by child development specialists, is not defined as such by many low-status families and can be viewed as their means of binding children to the haven of the family group, where they will be valued. Efforts to teach middle-class child rearing practices are often met with passive resistance. This would suggest that health and welfare personnel attempting to modify such behaviors are treating the symptom rather than the problem.

Regardless of the larger politico-cultural causal factors, however, disturbances in the families of the very poor are perceived as problems to be dealt with by a variety of community institutions. In the absence of any systemic reforms in the economic-social system, the available remedies (such as shelters for battered women, psychological counseling, foster care for children) entail the risk that families will be dissolved and invididuals with little access to economic resources will be set adrift from the very family systems that have been their strength and protection.

It is in firsthand accounts of the ordinary lives of individuals, in oral histories and biographies, that one often encounters a more sympathetic treatment of Appalachian female character. In studies of this type, Appalachian women are likely to be portrayed as proud and decent with a natural dignity (Kahn 1972; Lewis, Selfridge et al. 1986). The realities of their uncompromising environment and the economic exploitation of their families may have led to feelings of frustration and anger but have also motivated efforts to resist future exploitation (Kahn 1972). The women are noted to show "courage, humor and strength in the face of formidable odds" (Smith 1986). Although it is the nature of this type of literature to feature the positive traits of the subjects, these reports also demonstrate that the central role for women is as the protector of the emotional well-being of the family (whether that be the nuclear family, the single-parent family, or the larger family of humankind). These women have been called upon to comfort and cater to men who have faced failure and humiliation in the larger world. They have attempted to defend their children against the slurs and prejudices of those who have superior economic positions. They have banded together to protest the industrial insults to their families and their environment. But the documents also make it clear that this role expectation—to be a strong, emotionally sup-

portive woman—has its own price, paid in fatigue, emotional deple-
tion, depression, and frustrated anger that can result in periodic
emotional dysfunction.

SELF-PERCEPTIONS OF APPALACHIAN WOMEN

The perspectives of low-status women discussed up to this point may
seem, at times, contradictory. Are they unsophisticated hedonists and
apathetic drudges or stoic protectors of the family? The wide variety
of reported perceptions are probably attributable to the range of persons and behaviors encountered by the observers, the level of observation dictated by different professional disciplines, and the
underlying ideological positions that structure the studies. It is certainly feasible that much of what has been reported is true for some
part of the population under discussion. But, there is a further dimension that can be added to enhance an understanding of the social
world of low-status women in Appalachia. This dimension can be
derived from an analysis of the ways the women describe and explain
themselves. For the women under discussion are more than products
of their social context or the sum of their psychological characteristics;
they are creative actors within their social sphere.

This approach differs methodologically from the more strictly nar-
rative methods of oral histories. It entails the analysis of women's
stories, using the grounded theory method developed by Glaser and
Strauss (1967), to discover the embedded categories of meaning in
their revealed social world. The possibilities of this approach for understanding low-status women will be demonstrated in the following
illustrations taken from a series of informal interviews, conducted by
the author, with eighteen rural women over a five-month period.

The study was conducted in an East Tennessee county, hereafter
referred to by the pseudonym Clark County. Clark County is essentially rural; the majority (75%) of the population lives outside of its
two small towns, and 87% are native Tennesseans. The county's
largely unspoiled environment consists of scenic mountains, narrow
river valleys, and rolling, rocky farmland. Although the county lacks
major mineral deposits, it has a wealth of timber that is still being
harvested. The industrial park in the county seat flourished during a
brief boom in the early 1970s, but there has been a steady attrition of
small industries out of the county. Unemployment is endemic, av-
eraging over 20% in the winter months. The tourist industry in nearby
areas provides temporary summer employment, usually consisting of

minimum wage jobs in service occupations for women. Almost one quarter (23.68%) of the families in the county have incomes below the poverty level (U.S. Bureau of the Census 1982) and are receiving food stamps (Tennessee Advisory Commission on Intergovernmental Relations 1985). Only 40% of the residents graduated from high school.

The subjects of this study were participants in a local child development program, which serves children under four. The study participants were Appalachian born and raised. Excluded from the study were women experiencing current, severe family or legal problems.

The eighteen informants, all mothers, ranged in age from 21 to 67; slightly more than half of them were in their twenties. They represented fourteen different households. Only four women lived in traditional nuclear families, six households contained three generations of family members, and seven households were headed by women, representative of the varied family composition so seldom noted in Appalachian studies. Three women had never married, seven were divorced, two had separated, and one was widowed. This group of women had a fertility rate considerably higher than the national average of fewer than two pregnancies per woman. The women under 30 had averaged 3 pregnancies apiece while, the older women had on the average 6.6 pregnancies. (These figures exclude the subject in her sixties who at 20 pregnancies had more than double the pregnancies of anyone else in the group.) Although the younger women had stayed in school a few years longer than the older women, only one had graduated from high school and one had a GED.

In Appalachia, as in the rest of the United States, female-headed households are over represented in poverty groups. In the southern Appalachian region, which includes all of Tennessee's Appalachian counties, 11% of the non-female-headed families live in poverty, compared to 36.8% of the female-headed families with children (Tickamyer and Tickamyer 1987). All the households in the study under discussion were below the rural poverty level. Nuclear family groups, however, were more likely to have earned income than female-headed households. The majority of the families existed on some combination of Aid to Dependent Children, Social Security, or VA benefits supplemented by food stamps. Few of the informants had ever worked outside the home and belonged to the class of women described by Petchesky (1983) as being "the high fertility, low-labor-force participation group . . . who never or hardly ever work outside the home and are married to working-class men or receiving welfare" (p. 231).

The following self-descriptions were not necessarily planned or deliberate statements about self. That is, the informants were not asked to describe themselves nor did they say, "This is what I'm like." Rather, the descriptions were embedded in the context of stories about life events and emerged during data analysis. A few contextual facts about each informant will be appended to their self-definitions to provide a context for the reader and to illustrate the ways in which the women also fit into descriptive categories developed through the use of alternative perspectives discussed earlier.

These women have experienced multiple stresses in their lives. Chronic economic hardships have affected their health, their marital relationships, and the life chances of the children they have nurtured. They had a high probability of being born into families that were fractured by divorce or the early death of a parent; some of them have been the victims of sexual abuse and physical violence. Yet their self-images display resiliency and resourcefulness.

One self-perception which emerges is that these are women who persevere. Perseverance is highlighted in stories about continuing to tackle a problem in the face of apparent failure or in doing what is needed despite multiple obstacles. Lorraine keeps trying to learn how to swim despite her fear of water. At age 56, she keeps going back to swimming class each summer and doesn't plan to give up trying. She is raising two grandchildren and her own children move in and out of her housing project apartment.

Ida persevered and is proud of it. She remembers her struggle after her husband left her with 15 children to raise and little income. Five of the children came down with pneumonia. She nursed them back to health at home and even the doctor complimented her efforts. Ida accomplished her child-rearing tasks in the early 1950s while receiving $91 a month from AFDC and before Medicaid benefits were available.

A second image which emerges is that of hard-working women. Hard work was defined by the informants as physical labor done outside of the house. It might entail physical upkeep of the house and property (fixing the roof, painting the house, mowing the large yard), or actually building a home. Women in female-headed households taking responsibility for the care and upkeep of their residences were likely to express this type of self-definition.

A less traditional way of defining themselves as workers was expressed by two of the women in their twenties. They felt the happiest when able to work outside the home. Here it isn't the nature of the work that is important (one subject had been a nurse's aide, another a motel maid) but the invigorating feeling that accompanies being employed away from home. The self-definition as a worker thus takes precedence over identification in homemaking roles. The informants believe working in the community enhances their performance in the home. These statements were made by Jane and Barbara (both married to men from outside of the area), who have three and four children, respectively. Both husbands have periodic difficulty finding employment. Barbara and her family had to camp out in a garage recently for several months after she had a new baby and they were down on their luck. Jane and her family spent the coldest winter in recent memory, four years ago, in an uninsulated, converted bus.

A third way in which these informants characterized themselves was as worldly women. The importance of access to experiences in developing positive self-concepts is demonstrated by the following two women. Other informants had confided that they felt physically unwell when they left their county; however, when they were forced to do this over time (as when they had to take a handicapped child to repeated medical appointments in a nearby urban area) their anxiety abated. Low-status Appalachian women are not alone in harboring fears of the bigger world outside of the known perimeter of home and neighborhood.

Two women described their ability to have anxiety-free interactions in the larger social world outside of home and family and even outside of the local community. They credit this ability to the experience they gained through living and/or traveling to places outside of Tennessee. Ida attributes her superior knowledge of the world to living in a mill-town in North Carolina during her childhood, 60 years ago, while Lorraine, after separating from her husband, has traveled on her own to visit relatives over 300 miles away.

In a fourth means of self-definition, some women perceived themselves as independent minded. This is defined by one woman as not taking orders from others. True to the Appalachian nonconfrontational style, this is not done in defiance. In Barbara's definition, an independent-minded woman knows how to bargain to gain her own way. Her husband, who is practically illiterate, had been against her reading so many books. Barbara told him she'd give up the books if he'd give up something of comparable value, but they could not decide on what that something would be. Her husband finally just gave up his demand, and recently he even bought her a whole box of books at the flea market. An independent-minded woman also knows when to compromise and when to keep her mouth shut, so she can continue to have her own way. Barbara is determined to discipline her children her way despite the criticism of her husband and father-in-law, so she just listens to what they say, smiles to herself and does as she pleases, since she spends most of her time alone with the children. Barbara contrasts this type of independent-minded woman with "women libbers who want to be like a man." She is defining her style of being her own person, and regardless of feminist critiques of this style, Barbara perceives it as a way of controlling her social reality.

A fifth self-definition, in contrast to the description of women in this status group as present oriented, is that of planner. Present behaviors are justified by the women interviewed based on their projections of the behavior outcomes. They describe themselves as either being concerned with behavior outcomes or as convinced that certain outcomes are tied to specific behaviors.

Jane brought this up when she reflected on why she remained a virgin until she married (her own mother hadn't married the fathers of her several children). Jane said, at first, that she hadn't been much interested in boys and romance, but then added that she always was one to worry about the future and "what was down the road." Nora has a firm idea about how she should train her grandchildren to act when they are in autos, based on her assumptions of the possible consequences to children who are rowdy and disturb the driver. Nora is an illiterate grandmother, who protects her two young grandchildren by keeping them in their cribs much of the day (to the despair of her child development worker). Barbara chooses not to interfere in the disputes among her four children so the younger ones will learn not to allow older or larger children to bully them. An outside observer might assume that Barbara is a lazy or uncaring mother, or apathetic about the behavior of her children, unless enlightened by her view of her parenting priorities.

Finally, some of the informants considered themselves women with backbone. The ability to turn one's life around, to bring victory out of disaster, is an all-American story, featured regularly in our Sunday magazines. Such stories appear no more miraculous than the turnaround demonstrated by two women in this study. Both had spent years of their lives in desperate marriages filled with abuse and neglect. If interviewed during those years, each would have qualified for Polansky et al.'s (1972) study of the apathy-futility syndrome.

One of the women described the change in her life as the process of getting backbone. Backbone, as she defines it, is the inner feeling that you can stand up to life and you won't let anyone beat you down.

Lorraine said she used to "hump up to life," just taking the blows as they came but now she can stand up tall. For more than 15 years, she accepted her husband's opinion that she was dumb and, thus, no one would want to employ her. She credits her growing hatred of her philandering spouse as the means of her emancipation and new sense of selfhood.

Reena conveyed the same substantial feeling when she talked about her passage from a beaten, helpless wife to the confident, competent woman she is today. Backbone seems to be something one has to find within oneself and significantly both of these women suffered endless indignities before they initiated self-change. Reena had lived in abject poverty with her abusive husband and five children, begging for food because he had stolen the food stamps. When community agencies intervened and she faced the loss of her children, Reena began to change and, with the aid of a human service agency's homemaker, has made a new life for herself. Reena ultimately left her husband, although she continues to live in fear of him.

The positive self-images of women in this study often seem incongruent with some of the more visible aspects of their lives. Many of the older women appear lined and careworn beyond their years. Even the younger women show the beginnings of chronic dental problems that distract from their appearances. Their clothing is secondhand and their haircuts may be shapeless and unflattering. Yet, their self-definitions demonstrate that to evaluate them only in terms of these appearances or the roles they enact within their families and social strata does them an injustice.

IMPLICATIONS FOR MENTAL HEALTH PLANNING

The prevalent images of low-status women in the social science literature and the contrast with women's own self-perceptions suggest the following implications for those concerned with mental health issues.

Pertinent to the lives of individual rural low-status women is the nature of change in their social world. More of them are finding themselves single parents with little expectation of economic assistance except from government programs. Faced with a life of poverty, some women search for alternatives, but their socialization and education have not prepared them to enter competitive job markets or even given them the skills of interacting with the world outside the circle of their immediate acquaintances. The question to be addressed is how to assist these women to broaden their horizons and opportunities while avoiding the "make them like us" approach of the nineteenth-century missionary women.

The social and economic dependency of low-status women leaves them few choices when they are faced with failing or violent marriages or separation and divorce. While individual or group counseling may help them weather the immediate emotional stress, it cannot prevent them from falling even deeper into poverty. The women would benefit from access to jobs (paying better than minimum wage and carrying health and retirement benefits) and the supportive systems necessary to their employment, affordable day care and reliable transportation. Job-training programs keyed to the available job markets could enhance their opportunities. In this respect, the resources valuable to women are little different in Appalachia than elsewhere in the United States. But to what degree is it practical to focus on the needs of individual women in light of the overall economic picture in the region? In this respect, as in many others, the well-being of low-status women is inexorably tied to planning that will affect the future economic development of Appalachia.

Low-status women are frequently sent as family representatives to negotiate with community agencies for resources needed to meet family needs. As such, they easily become the focus of services that attempt to intervene in the family and ensure its adherence to community norms in terms of health and child care and protection. Intervention programs then can become a source of stress for low-status women and can reinforce their isolation and burden of responsibility. Transportation and child care are often cited as the barriers that prevent agencies from developing the type of self-help groups that have proven beneficial to women in urban areas. Such barriers must be addressed in planning any program for rural women.

Finally, the continued stereotyping of low-status women must be challenged. Social scientists and mental health professionals can play a role in discrediting stereotyped images, in communicating to the larger community the complexity of the low-status woman's social world, and in ensuring that her voice will be heard.

REFERENCES

Ball, R.A. 1968. A poverty case: The analgesic subculture of the southern Appalachians. *American Sociological Review* 33:885-95.

Beaver, P.D. 1976. Symbols and social organization in an Appalachian community. Ph.D. diss., Duke University, Durham, N.C.

Beaver, P.D. 1986. *Rural community in the Appalachian South*. Lexington: University Press of Kentucky.

Cavender, A. 1981. An ethnographic inquiry into social identity, social stratification, and premature school withdrawal in a rural Appalachian school. Ph.D. diss., University of Tennessee, Knoxville.

Coles, R. 1971. *Children of crisis*, vol. 2, *Migrants, sharecroppers, mountaineers*. Boston: Little, Brown.

Fisher, S.L. 1977. Folk culture or folk tale: Prevailing assumptions about the Appalachian personality. In *An Appalachian symposium: Essays written in honor of Cratis D. Williams*, 14-27. Boone, N.C.: Appalachian State University Press.

Fitchen, J.M. 1981. *Poverty in rural America: A case study*. Boulder, Colo.: Westview Press.

Gaventa, J. 1980. *Power and powerlessness: Quiescence and rebellion in an Appalachian valley*. Urbana: University of Illinois Press.

Glaser, B.G., and A.L. Strauss. 1967. *The discovery of grounded theory: Strategies for qualitative research*. Chicago: Aldine.

Heller, P.L., and G.M. Quesada. 1977. Rural familism: An interregional analysis. *Rural Sociology* 42(2):220-39.

Hicks, G.L. 1976. *Appalachian valley*. New York: Holt, Rinehart, and Winston.

Kahn, K. 1972. *Hillbilly women*. New York: Avon.

Kaplan, B.H. 1971. *Blue Ridge: an Appalachian community in transition*. Morgantown, W.Va.: Office of Research and Development, Appalachian Center, University of West Virginia.

Keefe, S.E., U.M.L. Reck, and G.G. Reck. 1985. Family and education in southern Appalachia. Paper presented at the annual meeting of the Appalachian Studies Conference, Berea, Ky.

Lewis, H.M., and E.E. Knipe. 1978. The colonialism model: The Appalachian case. In *Colonialism in modern America: The Appalachian case*, eds. H.M. Lewis, L. Johnson and D. Askins, 9-31. Boone, N.C.: The Appalachian Consortium Press.

Lewis, H.M., S. Kobak, and L. Johnson. 1978. Family, religion and colonialism in central Appalachia. In *Colonialism in modern America: The Appalachian case*, eds. H.M. Lewis, L. Johnson, and D. Askins, 113-139. Boone, N.C.: The Appalachian Consortium Press.

Lewis, H.M., L. Selfridge, J. Merrifield, S. Thrasher, L. Perry, and C. Honneycutt, eds. 1986. *Picking up the pieces: Women in and out of work in the rural South*. New Market, Tenn.: Highlander Research and Educational Center.

Looff, D.H. 1971. *Appalachia's children: The challenge of mental health*. Lexington: University Press of Kentucky.

Parenstedt, E. 1965. A comparison of the child-rearing environment of upper-lower and very low-income class families. *American Journal of Orthopsychiatry* 35:89-98.

Petchesky, R.P. 1983. Reproduction and class divisions among women. In *Class, race and sex: The dynamics of control*, eds. A. Swerdlow and H. Lessinger, 221-241. Boston: G.K. Hall.

Photiadis, J.D. N.d. *An overview of the processes of social transition in rural Appalachia*. Morgantown: Office of Research and Development, Center for Extension and Continuing Education, West Virginia University.

Photiadis, J.D. 1970. Rural southern Appalachia and mass society. In *Change in rural Appalachia: Implications for action programs*, ed. J.D. Photiadis and H.K. Schwarzweller, 5-22. Philadelphia: University of Pennsylvania Press.

Photiadis, J.D. 1986. *Community and family change in rural Appalachia*. Morgantown: West Virginia University Center for Extension and Continuing Education.

Polansky, N.A., R.A. Borgman, and C. De Saix. 1972. *Roots of futility*. San Francisco: Jossey-Bass.

Schwarzweller, H.K., J.S. Brown, and J.J. Mangalam. 1971. *Mountain families in transition: A case study in Appalachian migration*. University Park: Pennsylvania State University Press.

Smith, B.E. 1986. Women in the South: Economic survival. In *Picking up the pieces: Women in and out of work in the rural South*, eds. H.M. Lewis, L. Selfridge, J. Merrifield, S. Thrasher, L. Perry, and C. Honeycutt, 4-5. New Market, Tenn.: Highlander Research and Education Center.

Stephenson, J.B. 1968. *Shiloh: A mountain community*. Lexington: University Press of Kentucky.

Tennessee Advisory Commission on Intergovernmental Relations. 1985. *Fiscal, economic and social profiles of county areas in Tennessee*.

Tickamyer, A.R., and C. Tickamyer. 1987. Gender, family structure, and poverty in central Appalachia. In *The land and economy of Appalachia: Proceedings from the 1986 conference on Appalachia*, 80-90. Lexington: Appalachian Center, University of Kentucky.

U.S. Bureau of the Census. 1982. *Census of population: 1980, general, social and economic characteristics*. Washington, D.C.: U.S. Government Printing Office.

Walls, D.S., and D.B. Billings. 1977. The sociology of southern Appalachia. *Appalachian Journal* 4:131-44.

Weeks, J.S. 1980. Is the mountain woman unique? A debate. In *The Appalachian woman: Images and essence*, ed. P.B. Cheek, 22-26. Mars Hill, N.C.: Council on Appalachian Women.

Weller, J.E. 1965. *Yesterday's people: Life in contemporary Appalachia*. Lexington: University of Kentucky Press.

6

The Social Context of "Nerves" in Eastern Kentucky

EILEEN VAN SCHAIK

Are you a woman? Do you understand the meaning of "shattered nerves?"
Are you tortured with every form of suffering? Aches in the back and side
and head? Do you get nearly beside yourself over trifles? Does your face grow
thin and haggard? Are you completely discouraged and tired of life?[1]

The history of women's health chronicles the cultural construction of illness after illness—neurasthenia, hysteria, nervous prostration, and chlorosis to name just a few—that embodied the conflicts and contradictions experienced by women as they strove to make their place in the changing family and society of the late nineteenth and early twentieth century patriarchal, capitalist, industrial order (Brumberg 1984; Duffin 1978; Ehrenreich and English 1978; Figlio 1983; Smith-Rosenberg and Rosenberg 1984; Wood 1984). Dissatisfied and distressed women of the middle and upper classes consulted the growing number of male physicians who specialized in female disorders. For these women "It was acceptable, even fashionable to retire to bed with 'sick headaches,' 'nerves,' and a host of other mysterious ailments" (Ehrenreich and English 1973, p. 18). Women of all classes, including working-class and poor women, medicated themselves with patent medicines and consulted popular home readers or "doctor books" that advised them on the care of their feminine nervous systems (Ehrenreich and English 1978; Thomas 1983). Patent medicine advertisements regularly linked nervous disorders with the female reproductive system (Thomas 1983). Lydia Pinkham, for example, cautioned schoolgirls, shop girls, and society women that they were in danger of "nervous prostration, excitability, fainting spells, most likely organic diseases of the uterus or womb, and many other distressing female troubles" (Hechtlinger 1970, p. 77).

Writing in 1895, Dr. Mary Putnam Jacobi observed that for women, "it is considered natural and almost laudable to breakdown under all conceivable varieties of strain. . . . Constantly considering their nerves, urged to consider them by well-intentioned but short-sighted advisors, they pretty soon become nothing but a bundle of nerves" (quoted in Ehrenreich and English 1973, p. 108).

Nearly one hundred years later women are still considering their nerves. Late-twentieth-century women continue to experience their conflicts and anxieties as illness, especially as "nervous" or "mental illness." Women today receive more prescriptions for psychotropic drugs than men and they receive more outpatient psychotherapy (Clarke 1983; Riessman 1983). From Lydia Pinkham to Valium, women have been encouraged to call their dissatisfactions illness and to remedy them through the use of medications. In the late twentieth century, nerves are reported among clusters of impoverished and socially neglected women.

Today, practitioners in eastern Kentucky observe that many of their female patients seek treatment for their nerves and generally expect to receive "nerve pills" for their complaints (Flannery 1982). Often these patients report that a previous physician told them that their symptoms are due to nerves. A thorough medical history, according to Flannery, generally reveals the complex and difficult social situations that perpetuate their symptoms. In a study of a Newfoundland fishing village, Davis (1982, 1983) found that 90% of the women complain of nerves and generally rely on nerve pills for relief. The majority of the women in childbearing years whom Harrison (1982) met in a mountain community in El Salvador complain of nervios and receive psychotropic drugs for their symptoms.

Nerves are reported by men as well as women among Appalachian populations (Arny 1955; Dornbran n.d.; Friedl 1978; Leighton and Cline 1968; Ludwig 1982; Ludwig and Forrester 1981, 1982; Mabry 1964; Wiesel and Arny 1952) and among some cultural groups in Central America (Barlett and Low 1980; Low 1981; Low and Hammer 1983). It is possible, however, that the experience of nerves differs for men from that of women. Women as a group experience their social world differently from men as a group (Ferguson 1984). Their roles as daughters, sisters, wives, and mothers differ from the family roles of men as do the roles available to them in the larger public world. Women's encounters with others and their knowledge of themselves are institutionally and linguistically structured in ways that differ from those of men.[2] The long standing practice of medicalizing the conflicts and contradictions in women's lives is one example of the differently structured experiences of women. This paper presents an account of nerves as offered by women who voice the complaint and argues that the social context is a critical component of nerves.[3]

METHODOLOGY

The following description of nerves is based on interviews with eight women from eastern Kentucky who identify themselves as having nerves.[4] Six were interviewed in a community clinic in an eastern Kentucky county and two were interviewed in their homes after an initial meeting in the clinic. A short list of open-ended questions, based on those developed by Kleinman (1980) for eliciting explanatory models of illness, was used to guide the interviews and all interviews were tape-recorded after obtaining the informant's permission. The women, identified by pseudonyms, range in age from 14 to 82 years. As suggested by their life histories, all are of lower socioeconomic status. A brief introduction to each woman is followed by a discussion of her symptoms and course of nerves, the woman's etiological explanations for nerves, and the role of professional medicine in constructing nerves.

THE INFORMANTS

Flora is an eighty-two-year-old widow whose husband died many years ago of Hodgkins disease. Flora's husband had two children whom she helped raise; however, one has died and she does not see the other. Although a niece has invited Flora to live with her, she declines to do so because her niece is already responsible for the care of an elderly parent. Flora lives alone, does her own housework, and raises a vegetable garden, although she tires with prolonged digging and walking uphill.

Dorothy is a sixty-four-year-old wife and mother of 11 children. Her husband, a retired coal miner, suffers from a serious lung condition and some form of mental deterioration that Dorothy attributes to his many years of heavy drinking.

One son, who is disabled by a heart condition, lives with Dorothy and her husband, whereas the other children live throughout Kentucky, Indiana, Ohio, and Texas. Dorothy worries a great deal about her sons and daughters who work in hazardous occupations, live far away, and not infrequently experience illnesses or automobile accidents on mountain roads. Dorothy is one of five children and left school at the age of nine to help raise her brothers and sisters when her mother died.

Marie is about fifty years old. Her first husband left her with two small sons, whom she raised with the help of her grandmother. Subsequently she cared for her grandmother, who by then was blind and ill, until the woman died. When Marie's sons were nine and fourteen years old, she married her present husband, who, she says, has been a good father to her boys.

Marie's oldest son died fourteen years ago of leukemia. Marie's youngest son, his wife, and their child are daily visitors in her home. Marie currently is raising three young nieces, one of whom lives with her; the other two live next door with their father. Marie, in addition, worries about her present husband, who suffers from a seizure disorder, her brother and sister, both of whom suffer from nerves, and her elderly mother. Pointing to the houses clustered around hers, Marie identifies the homes of her mother, aunt, sister, two brothers, and son, saying "It's all [my] people" and admitting that there is a "lot of worry" to having a large family.

Clara, who is forty-two years old, has been married for twenty-eight years and is the mother of four children. According to Clara, her husband has been drinking heavily for the last eighteen years. Although she left him, six and a half years ago, to move to Chicago, where two of her daughters live, Clara returned to Kentucky after losing her welfare and food stamp benefits. Her only son left home two years ago, and she does not know where he is now. Her fourteen-year-old daughter lives with Clara and her husband and attends a "special education" program. Some years ago, Clara's own parents and her older and younger brother died, all within 11 months of each other.

Stella, who married at fourteen years of age, is forty years old and observes "I've been married all my life." Her first husband died within the last four years, and she is currently divorcing her second husband. Stella has a twenty-four-year-old son, who works in the coal mines and visits her daily, and a twenty-year-old daughter, who telephones daily and visits about three times a week. Although their relationships appear settled now, Stella suffered a great deal several years ago, when her son served time in the penitentiary and her daughter, then fourteen years of age, underwent an abortion.

Stella worked for some time as a beautician before she suffered a "stroke." She is now employed in a less demanding job in a small store that pays her two dollars an hour. Her mother lives nearby and assists Stella financially.

Betty is a thirty-eight-year-old woman whose first husband was killed in the coal mines. For most of the twenty-three years of this marriage, according to Betty, he drank heavily, went out with other women, beat her, and squandered their money. Living in Maryland and Ohio, Betty worked in hotels, restaurants, and textile plants "to buy my kids shoes." Betty has two sons, one twenty and the other eighteen years old, and a fourteen-year-old daughter. Her sons have been in jail numerous times and Betty was threatened with loss of custody of her daughter, who was repeatedly delinquent earlier in her adolescence. Betty's older son now works in the coal mines and her daughter recently married and settled in the area. Betty's own childhood was marked by poverty and the illness of her father, a disabled miner. She quit school and began working to help support her family at 15 years of age. Betty's second marriage was a failure, lasting only a few months.

Ann is twenty years old and lived in Michigan for several years before returning to Kentucky. According to Ann, her first husband drank heavily and beat her. Their marriage ended some time after Ann gave birth to a hydrocephalic infant, who died within a few hours. Ann's second marriage, of 16 months duration, is troubled by disagreements between Ann and her in-laws, who wish the couple to live with them. Neither Ann nor her husband, a coal miner, is employed at present, although Ann reports that she would like to work if she could find a job in the area.

Shirley is only fourteen years old, and both of her parents are deceased. Her mother died five months ago and her father died five years ago. Shirley claims that her father treated her "mean" all of her life and refused to support her mother and the children. She has seven brothers and sisters, several of whom are married and living in other counties or states. She complains about living with her grandmother, who she claims does not want her, and is temporarily staying with an eighty-year-old neighbor woman, providing assistance in the house and earning a small income. The clinic staff confirm that Shirley has been treated poorly, sent from place to place to live, and is not wanted by her grandmother.

Together the lives of these eight women reflect a variety of responses to the struggle for subsistence in the coal-mining economy of eastern Kentucky. Their fathers, husbands, or sons mine coal, experience unemployment, and suffer debilitating chronic diseases. As women faced with the need to support their families, they find even fewer employment opportunities than the men. Together with their families some migrated temporarily to northern and eastern states seeking employment. A few began the struggle for subsistence in their childhood, leaving school to raise their siblings or to earn money for their families. All work in their homes, keeping house, raising gardens, and caring for children and aged or ill family members. All but the youngest two have children or stepchildren and have spent a good part of their lives providing them with material necessities, caring for them, and worrying over their well-being. Some of these women live alone now, their only source of support being their children or their own mothers. From their individual experiences a common theme emerges, which is aptly stated by Dorothy, "I seen hard all my life, even in my young days I seen hard." These women identify the signs and symptoms of distress that arise during their lives as nerves.

"IT FEELS LIKE A FEAR RIGHT IN YOUR FLESH"

In the words of these women, nerves are experienced as feelings of nervousness and aggravation, anger, impatience, fearfulness, and depression. Five of them state that feeling nervous is one component of nerves, and two of them frequently refer to being "nervous and aggravated." Clara describes the day before her interview as an example: she got up in the morning so "nervous and aggravated" with herself that she felt like "pulling [her] hair out." She was "so nervous" she "liked to croaked and what caused it [she] couldn't tell you." For these women, the experience of nerves includes a heightened sensitivity to irritations and worries. Clara explains that "little old things set you off. Don't take much to set you off if you got 'em [nerves] bad." Stella describes her nerves by saying "I'm just a nervous person, sometimes worse than others, a lot of times I worry more than I should. I'm a worrier."

Becoming angry, cursing, and calling names are among the symptoms of nerves identified by four individuals. Clara describes occasions when she wants "to hurt something or other, take my spite out on something or other." She takes a "nerve pill" at such times and finds work to do, often chopping wood. Three of the women interviewed associate feeling fearful with nerves. For Marie and Ann, these fears focus on their health and the possibility of dying. Marie expresses apprehension about what will become of her family if she is unable to care for them. Ann admits that her imagination "runs away" causing her to be easily frightened by the slightest sign of illness. At such times, Ann wants to see a physician immediately and, if there is no money for gas or no one willing to drive her, she becomes convinced that she will die and no one will care.

Flora identifies her nerves as "depression" and describes the feeling this way: "Seems like things are not a joy to you, your life is a burden or something. It's a bad feeling. It seems like it just takes the joy out of your life. You don't enjoy things like you would if they weren't bothering you." Flora believes that if her nerves were better she would enjoy her work but as she feels now, she "makes" herself do her cleaning, gardening, and "one thing and another," which recently included some painting. Despite these activities, Flora, who suffers from multiple chronic illnesses, complains that she "lays around" and sleeps too much. Ann also complains of sleeping too much, stating that she sometimes sleeps from eleven in the evening until one in the afternoon and yet is so tired that she takes a nap later in the day. Unlike Flora, Ann does not complain of depression; instead she attributes her tiredness to "sitting around with nothing to do," pointing out that she cannot find employment and has no children.

All of these women complain of some form of physical agitation or restlessness associated with nerves. Three of them report trembling, shaking, and jerking all over as a sign of nerves. In addition, these informants observe that they cannot hold onto things, cannot tolerate being still, and must be going all of the time. Agitation and restlessness may be relieved by finding something to do, going for a walk, or driving a car. Four informants describe the urge to open doors, to get out, or to run away during episodes of nerves. Betty explains that during earlier episodes of nerves she could not tolerate being in the same room with her husband, and to this day, she cannot tolerate a closed door.

Observing that when her nerves are bad she cannot tolerate waiting, Flora describes the feeling as "a going in me" or as "something in the flesh, something's got you and you cannot get away from it. It feels like a fear right in your flesh." That nerves are experienced "in the flesh" is also suggested by three informants who complain of itching, especially on their hands and feet, their back, or simply "all over."

Both Marie and Ann associate an increased heart rate with nerves. Marie did not initially believe that her symptoms were due to nerves: "this" she told herself "is real." After being reassured by her physician that her heart is all right, receiving a prescription for phenobarbital, and switching to decaffeinated coffee, however, Marie finds "I've not been bothered with it no more, it's never bothered me again, so evidently it's been my nerves." In addition, Marie reports that her "blood is a little high" and that her physician attributes this to nerves as well. Dorothy also reports that her blood pressure goes up when she is upset and, because she is easily upset, elevated blood pressure is a chronic problem for which she sees her physician once a month.

Four of these women report gastrointestinal complaints or weight loss associated with nerves. Betty reports that she cannot eat during episodes of nerves and describes periods of prolonged vomiting associated with nerves. Betty, who also complains of choking and inability to swallow, reports that she loses weight during such episodes and uses her weight as an indicator of the state of her nerves, citing weight gains for those times when her nerves are "calm" and weight loss whenever her nerves are at their worst. Stella reports dropping to 92 pounds during her first major episode with nerves, which resulted in hospitalization. She admits that today she often does not eat as she should, in part because she lives alone. Dorothy, on the other hand, finds that she eats more when she is nervous and states that she is overweight and finds it difficult to lose weight. She also reports that she develops diarrhea from rushing and becoming nervous. Shirley has been to the clinic several times with complaints of stomach pain, which she admits might be linked to nerves.

Betty and Dorothy complain that they are unable to sleep because of their nerves. Ann "smothers"[5] and finds that her fears for her health increase at night; and Marie's rapid and irregular heart beat also is worse at night, causing her to pace the floor until it returns to normal and she can sleep. Nerves are accompanied by crying according to three women and, in Betty's case, by crying and screaming. Headaches, often severe, are signs of nerves for three individuals. Stella complains of feeling weak and lightheaded during "nervous spells," Shirley complains of dizziness, and Betty describes episodes of fainting or partial loss of consciousness that she attributes to nerves.

None of these women reports being unable to work or fulfill her usual responsibilities because of her nerves. Although most are unemployed, it is not due to a nerves-related disability. In fact, Betty recalls that her nerves were "steady" during those periods when both she and her husband were working outside the home, and Ann is convinced that her nerves would improve if she had a job, more to do, or a child to raise. These women do admit, however, to difficulty with certain tasks. Betty reports that she forgets what she is doing or where she has placed things when her nerves are bad. Stella gave up employment as a beautician because she becomes nervous when she tries to hurry, experiencing difficulty with her speech, and actually working more slowly.

In summary, the symptoms of nerves, as described by these women, include feelings of nervousness, anger, impatience, fearfulness, and depression, as well as physical agitation and restlessness, insomnia, crying, and a variety of somatic complaints including gastrointestinal disturbances, weight loss, increased heart rate, elevated blood pressure, "smothering," headaches, and "black outs." This broad and general array of complaints makes it difficult to identify a distinct cluster of symptoms specific to nerves.[6] Nerves appears to be an illness category linked with a number of general symptoms; at the same time, several illnesses share features or symptoms common to nerves.[7]

THERE IS NO "CASTING THEM OFF"

For most of these informants the range and severity of their symptoms change over time, diminishing for some, increasing for others. There seems to be no inevitable progression of symptoms among these women just as there is no distinctive set of symptoms specific to nerves. It appears, on the basis of their accounts, however, that nerves is a chronic condition marked by periods of remission or improvement alternating with acute episodes or crises.

Flora was first hospitalized for nerves during her husband's illness and was in "terrible shape" after his death twenty years ago. She received "the shocks" and was "some better" following her discharge from the hospital but her nerves "bothered [her] along." Ann reports improvement in her nerves over the years, stating that her nerves are bad now but were worse when she was married to her first husband who "really made [her] a nervous wreck." Ann attributes her nerves alternately to her husband's drinking, stating that she began drinking and taking nerve pills herself while married to him, and to the death of her infant, saying "that aggravated me a lot. I don't know, I might have got my nerve problem from that, worrying about it so much." Clara, on the other hand, reports that her nerves have deteriorated or "left" in the last six or seven years, becoming even worse in the last two years as her husband's drinking increased. Clara denies any difficulty with her nerves before her husband began drinking. She states, "It's all because of my husband, every bit of it lays on him, no way out of it; he's an alcoholic"; and she adds that her nerves were "steady" while she was rearing her children and had no "aggravations." Clara also blames her husband's drinking for her daughter's crying spells, which she interprets as a sign that her daughter's "nerves are wrecked."

Betty reports several acute episodes of nerves, during which she thought she was "going crazy," followed by periods of improvement in which her nerves were "steady." Betty states "What really caused me to be nervous was him [her husband] taking me through all that, and then all that with Jenny [her daughter]. I like to went crazy with Jenny." The nature of Betty's symptoms are unchanged from one episode to the next, as she herself recognizes. Describing the ordeals she suffered with her daughter, Betty states that she could see that she "was getting just like I was with him [her husband]."

Unresolved episodes of nerves can lead, according to these women, to nervous breakdowns sometimes requiring hospitalization, or to thoughts of suicide. Stella describes three distinct episodes with her nerves, each of which differed from the other, although each resulted in hospitalization. During the first episode, when she was hospitalized for extreme weight loss, Stella did not believe her physician when they attributed her symptoms to nerves. Now she says "There was nothing really, nothing wrong with me, you know, not nothing physical real wrong with me." During the second episode, which she refers to as a "breakdown," she remained at home with the phone off the hook and the doors locked, convinced that no one liked her and that she herself liked no one. At one point she considered shooting herself, had a gun, and believes that she would have done so had her daughter not arrived when she did. Stella improved after three weeks in the hospital and has not experienced a similar episode again. According to Stella, the third hospital admission was for a "stroke," although she reports that her physician attributed this illness to nerves as well. Stella currently experiences "nervous spells" but denies any further thoughts of suicide. Reflecting on the difficult years when her son and daughter were in trouble, Stella states that "started a whole of it [nerves]."

Shirley's account of an attempt to "kill" herself by taking eight "blood pressure" pills suggests the chronic nature of her nerves and the social isolation underlying her distress:

Well, just so many people calling me names, just running over me, treating me so dirty, I just got tired of it; I just wanted to kill myself. I figured that they [taking the pills] would do the trick and it didn't do no trick. So, ah, so if I get the chance again and they ah, start doing me the same way, I'll take 'em again. Cause I, Linda [her cousin] knows, I been treated like a dog all my life. She knows sometimes they'd do her the same way, her sisters do. And I know how she feels, cause people do me the same way. Like at school, up here at Green Mountain, none of them don't like me and Linda so that just gets all over my nerves. I just go plum nutty. And I can't, I just can't stand for people doing me that way, cause I been that way ever since I was born.

"THEY SAY PRESSURE AND STRAIN CAUSES IT"

The life histories of these women suggest that nerves occur at all stages of the life cycle and are frequently associated with crises in family life. Clara, Betty, and Ann directly attribute their nerves to their husbands' abuse of alcohol. For Betty, conflicts and worry over her children were coupled with her husband's drinking, whereas Ann associates the death of her infant with the strife of her first marriage. Dorothy, too, speaks of the distress of living with an alcohol-abusing husband and admits that she worries a great deal over her children as well. Stella, too, attributes her nerves, in part, to worry over her children.

Although the youngest and oldest women have neither husbands nor children, they attribute their nerves to grief and distress over family members. Flora suggests that the prolonged strain of her husband's illness and eventual death may be partially to blame for her nerves. Shirley attributes the onset of nerves to the mean-spirited behavior of her father and to his death early in her life. The recent death of her mother and the belief that she is unwanted and disliked by her family and members of her community contribute to Shirley's nerves today. Clara, too, speaks at length about the death of her parents and brothers and doubts that she will ever recover from the loss.

The strain of caring for and worrying about family members is reflected in Marie's response when asked why she and several members of her family have trouble with nerves: "Everybody's good to everybody; we're all real close. Sometimes I think we're too close 'cause something gets wrong with one of them and everybody's worrying." The stresses of family life are compounded for all of these women by the strains of poverty and limited opportunities for local employment for themselves or their families.

In addition to familial and economic crises, the daily details of family life make an already nerve-prone existence more difficult for these informants. Ann, for example, spends a good deal of time with her younger siblings and occasionally becomes "aggravated" by their continual requests to be played with and taken places. Marie, too, finds that the incessant chatter of her nieces, at times, makes her "so nervous." Both women secure some measure of quiet and calm by letting the children know that they are "getting" on their "nerves." Both Marie and Dorothy admit that fatigue from long days cooking, cleaning, and caring for others may contribute to their symptoms. Rushing to church for morning and evening services amidst cooking and attending to others makes Sundays especially trying for both women.

Reports of illness and chronic disease that accompany these accounts of family turmoil, poverty, and hard work reveal yet another feature of the context in which nerves occur. Flora states several times, "I know my nerves bothers me, but that's not all that's wrong," and goes on to discuss the numerous chronic illnesses—such as diabetes, chronic cystitis, indigestion and "heart trouble"—that interfere with her daily activities. Marie and Ann both identify worry over their health and fear of dying as aspects of their nerves. Betty complains of an "ulcerated stomach" and also explains that she underwent a hysterectomy for cancer after her daughter was born. Dorothy is diabetic and has a history of obesity, thyroid disorder, arthritis of the spine, and hypertension but associates only the hypertension with her nerves. Clara reports repeated episodes of bronchitis and pneumonia.

Speaking of the problems of those with nerves, Betty states, "You've got to have somebody to reach down a helping hand and help you," indicating a need for support that the other informants identify as well.[8] Today, Stella calls on a friend when she is having a "nervous spell" and needs to talk with someone. But she was not always able to do so. Stella suggests that her nerves may be caused, at least in part, by the fact that she "never did talk to nobody." She states, "I think what it was with me, I lived in my own world and I didn't let nobody in; I didn't tell nobody nothing." She adds, however, that people do not care; they have their own problems and, furthermore, there are some things one simply cannot tell others. Stella's mother, for example, still does not know that her granddaughter had an abortion several years ago; nor do Stella's friends know about the incident. Clara also expresses the idea that others are not readily available to listen to and support her, "They've got ten thousand other things to talk about," and she states that she cannot talk to her husband. Like many of the women, Flora suggests that the support of others may be beneficial for nerves. She states, "I guess I ought to get out and go places whether I feel like it or not, talk with people around about. It might help me some."

These interviews suggest that the accumulated distress of marital discord, family worries, grief, limited employment opportunities, financial insecurity, illness, and lack of support may at times be overwhelming for these individuals and result in symptoms of nerves or in acute episodes of nerves.[9] The remarks of several informants suggest that there is a threshold of distress beyond which nerves will give way. Repeatedly Shirley states "I can take so much," and Stella remarks "Things build up." Dorothy, with her eleven children, observes that "There is always something" or that it is "one thing after another."

Symptoms that develop in the wake of accumulated distress are attributed to nerves by these women. As a popular illness term, nerves provides an interpretive framework used to construct and socially validate a medical reality that takes into account the sources of distress and makes sense of the resulting symptoms (Good and Good 1984). The validity of the illness may be confirmed by seeking support from physicians, family, and friends, by the prescription of nerve pills and shots, and by hospitalization.

NERVE PILLS—"ANYBODY CAN TAKE 'EM"

Physicians, as reported by these women, frequently identify their patients' complaints as nerves and fill a vital role in providing reassurance and support to the individual. Four women in the present study state that their physician first told them that their symptoms are due to nerves.[10] Marie is relieved by the diagnosis of nerves provided by her physician and is reassured that she has no heart disease. Despite feeling "real bad" on Sunday, Marie has experienced no further symptoms with her heart since seeing her physician and states "I'm 100% better than I was. Just talking to her helped. She assured me. I believe I'm going to be all right now."

Professional counselors, as well as physicians, provide guidance and reassurance to individuals with nerves. For a time, Ann attended a county mental center, where she spent the day participating in various activities, playing games, and talking to the staff. Ann states that the program was helping her and that she only discontinued participation when her husband lost his job and they could no longer afford it.

In addition, all of these informants rely on medication to relieve symptoms of nerves. Throughout these interviews, the medication taken for nerves is most frequently referred to as "nerve pill(s)" even by those who also use the trade name for their medication.[11] Of those three informants who identify their pills by name, two have taken Valium and one is taking phenobarbital.

With the probable exception of 14-year-old Shirley, all of these women have been taking nerve pills intermittently for many years. Only Dorothy and Clara admit to currently using nerve pills on a regular basis to relieve their symptoms throughout the day and to ensure sleep at night. The other six women report taking nerve pills only when they need them, that is, in times of acute symptoms and distress not on a routine basis. Of those six women who use the pills only as needed, all but two mention concern with their habit-forming nature. Most report that they achieve a desired state of "calm" from the pills and do rest better at night. Stella and Shirley, however, state that nerve pills do little good for them and Ann complains that nerve pills make her feel drowsy, produce a tingling in her head, and cause her to chill. Because she is "even scared of them," nerve pills do little to relieve Ann's apprehensions about her physical condition or her fears of dying.

The general acceptance of nerve pills among the present informants is reflected in the words of Mrs. Jones, the eighty-year-old neighbor with whom Shirley was living at the time of her interview. Mrs. Jones recently gave Shirley a nerve pill when the latter was distressed by two reportedly drunken neighbor men who were harassing her and threatening to enter the house. When questioned further about the pill, Mrs. Jones replied "Anybody can take 'em. They're only two milligram." This incident also reflects the way in which the daily practices of individuals reproduce the cultural preference for medicalizing the distress of women; younger women learn from older women to identify the outcomes of social relationships as private experiences, and to take medication for the resulting distress.

In addition to nerve pills, the need for "shots" and hospitalization are indicators of the severity of nerves and validate the medical nature of the complaint for these informants. Marie received a "treatment of nine shots" during her breakdown several years ago. While hospitalized and already quite distraught over her husband's drinking and violent behavior, Dorothy received word that one of her sons had been injured. She reports that she was so upset she was given "shots" to calm her. Repeatedly in each account of a crisis, Betty states "they had to give me shots to bring me down off that."

Four of these women have been hospitalized for nerves or nervous breakdowns. In addition, both Dorothy and Betty report that, in the past, they or someone in their family requested that their physician hospitalize them for their nerves, only to be told "No, your problems will be there when you return, piling up." The physician's response suggests that she recognizes the difficult life circumstances associated with nerves and sees no solution in medical treatment. The physician nevertheless frequently offers the diagnosis of nerves.

A recent incident in which Betty disagrees with her physician's diagnosis of nerves illustrates the social origins of the complaint and demonstrates that aspects of the individual's social context, not her symptoms, are critical in identifying nerves. Betty's regular physician was not available a few weekends before the interview when Betty went to the emergency room of a local hospital with complaints of nausea and vomiting, chills, and fever and was admitted. The following Monday, Betty's physician found her in the hospital. Krowing, however, that Betty's youngest son recently left for Florida to avoid arrest in Kentucky, the physician identified Betty's problem as nerves and promptly discharged her from the hospital with instructions to return to the clinic that week. At the time of the interview, Betty still insists that her symptoms are due to flu or to an ulcerated stomach. Yet, given her long history of acute episodes of nerves associated with crises with her sons and daughter, often involving conflicts with the law, it appears that once again Betty suffers from nerves.

Betty's physician bases her diagnosis on certain aspects of Betty's social environment not on her symptoms. Were her physician not attuned to the realities of Betty's social environment, the symptoms might well suggest flu or ulcerated stomach. The diagnosis of nerves links social context and symptoms, yet even as the source of distress is tacitly recognized, the notion of illness is perpetuated by labeling the trouble *nerves*.

DISCUSSION: "THIS IS REAL"

The present description of nerves suggests that a broad range of general symptoms is linked to social distress through the popular illness term *nerves*. The daily lives of women voicing the complaint are characterized by continuous struggles to cope with the responsibilities of

family life in a context of poverty, restricted opportunities for employment, and limited sources of emotional and social support. The
cumulative effect of this struggle results in symptoms attributed to
nerves. These women seek support from physicians, family, and
friends. In addition, they take nerve pills, receive "shots," and occasionally are hospitalized for their nerves, all of which confirm the
medical reality of their complaint. The relationship between the symptoms of nerves and social distress is implicitly recognized by these
women and by their physicians.

As a popular term encompassing both physical and emotional
symptoms, *nerves* enjoys at least a limited medical respectability and
gives voice to women's anguish without confronting the social arrangements underlying their distress. The culture provides ample
lessons in identifying and labeling distress as *nerves*. Women as young
as fourteen are given medication to relieve the distress they experience
in difficult social situations. Each woman interviewed knows at least
one other woman with nerves, often her mother or her daughter. The
widespread use of psychotropic drugs, readily identified by these
women as nerve pills, supports the belief that the nervous system,
not the social system, is at fault. Discovering that the difficult social
situations in which symptoms arise are beyond the scope of their
practice, physicians find it convenient to talk in terms of nerves,
thereby perpetuating the belief that the problem is medical after all.

In a culture that prefers to identify the social conflicts and inequities
experienced by women as private issues and the resulting signs of
distress as medical problems, women learn to recognize physical illness as legitimate and to discount their subjective experiences of the
social world as not "real." Marie's rapid heart rate convinced her that
her discomfort is "real," that is, physical and not imagined or psychological. Stella learned that her severe weight loss was due to her
state of mind, "there was nothing really, nothing wrong with me,
you know, not nothing physical real wrong with me." Marie, over-
whelmed by worry for her family and the responsibility of raising
three young girls, and Stella, isolated in her distress over her son's
imprisonment and her daughter's abortion, do not identify the social
and material origins of their distress. Turning to their physician for
validation of their experiences, Marie, Stella, and the others receive
pills and the reassurance that they are not "crazy," only "under a lot
of pressure and strain." In a similar manner, the hysteric and neuras-
thenic were consoled and medicated for their "disorders." Today,
nerves bespeaks the continuing cultural preference for individualizing

and medicalizing the distress of women who lack adequate social support for their familial and economic struggles.

NOTES

While writing this paper, I was supported by NIMH Research Training Grant 2 T32 MH15730-06. I would like to thank Susan Abbott for her guidance during the research on which this paper is based and Kathleen Blee for helpful comments during the preparation of this paper.

1. From the text of an advertisement for Dr. Greene's Nervura in *The Sacred Heart Review*, January 4, 1902, p. 902; quoted in Thomas 1983, p. 105.

2. See Horton (1984) for a discussion of culturally patterned differences in the illness complaints of men and women in Appalachia.

3. Previous studies that attempt to clarify the nature of nerves in Appalachia focus on symptoms and translate the term into conventional psychiatric nosology (Arny 1955; Ludwig and Forrester 1981, 1982; Wiesel and Arny 1952). Ludwig's (1982) attempt to provide a cultural interpretation of nerves is colored by his reliance on perjorative accounts (Caudill 1962; Looff 1971; Weller 1965) of Appalachian life and perpetuates stereotypes of passive, dependent, inadequate personalities, and cultural deprivation. Ludwig's sources are subjected to critical examination by Billings (1974), Coles (1971), Eller (1982), Fisher (1976), Lewis (1976), and Walls (1976).

4. These interviews are taken from a set of ten interviews conducted to obtain detailed phenomenological descriptions of nerves as experienced by those who report the complaint in eastern Kentucky (Van Schaik 1983).

5. *Smothering* is a popular term for shortness of breath or labored respirations. Flannery (1982) interprets the term in light of the prevalence of black lung disease and the history of oppression in Appalachia, where it is frequently heard.

6. The symptoms identified here are consistent with those reported elsewhere for eastern Kentucky (Dornbran n.d.; Flannery 1982; Ludwig and Forrester 1981, 1982; Ludwig 1982; Mabry 1964) and for Appalachian migrants in Ohio (Friedl 1978). The symptoms reported by Davis (1982, 1983) for Newfoundland are similar to those in the present study as are those reported for *nervios* in Central America (Barlett and Low 1980; Harrison 1982; Low 1981, 1984; Low and Hammer 1983).

7. See Fabrega (1970) on the specificity of folk illnesses.

8. An additional source of support is identified by Betty and Flora who speak of turning to the Lord for help with their nerves and the distress associated with them. Betty offers repeated testimonies to the help she received from the Lord as she faced the various crises in her life. Again and again, she states that the only "two people" she turned to in her crises were the "Good Lord" and her doctor. Betty explains the importance of both physicians and the Lord saying "God gives knowledge to doctors. . . . He can help . . . it takes both." The following advice offered by Betty suggests that physicians, friends, and the Lord are all necessary sources of support during a crisis with nerves: "get somebody, call a friend, have them to call a doctor, Doctor [her doctor]. Don't get so far gone that you would destroy yourself, commit suicide, hurt yourself. Get on the phone, talk to a friend, get a Bible, get a doctor, then start calling on the Lord."

9. Similarly, familial, social, and economic hardships are associated with nerves in Newfoundland (Davis 1982, 1983) and with *nervios* in Costa Rica (Barlett and Low 1980;

Low 1981, 1984; Low and Hammer 1983) and El Salvador (Harrison 1982). Low (1981, 1984) reports that physicians in urban Costa Rica recognize *nervios* as a clue to family or economic problems and direct their attention to the social context in which the symptoms develop.

10. Dornbran (n.d.), Low (1981, 1984), Ludwig (1982), and Ludwig and Forrester (1981) also report that physicians use the term *nerves* (or *nervios*) in discussions with their patients. This occurs despite the fact that when presented with the complaint some physicians find the term ambiguous and puzzling (Dornbran n.d.; Friedl 1978; Ludwig 1982; Mabry 1964).

11. Davis (1982, 1983), Dornbran (n.d.), Flannery (1982), Ludwig (1982), and Ludwig and Forrester (1981, 1982) also report a general reliance on "nerve pills" among those with nerves.

REFERENCES

Arny, M. 1955. My nerves are busted. *Mountain Life and Work* 3:24-29.

Barlett, P., and S. Low. 1980. *Nervios* in Rural Costa Rica. *Medical Anthropology* 4:523-59.

Billings, D. 1974. Culture and poverty in Appalachia: A theoretical discussion and empirical analysis. *Social Forces* 53:130-38.

Brumberg, J.J. 1984. Chlorotic girls, 1870-1920: A historical perspective on female adolescence. In *Women and health in America*, ed. J.W. Leavitt, 186-95. Madison: University of Wisconsin Press.

Caudill, H. 1962. *Night comes to the Cumberlands*. Boston: Little, Brown.

Clarke, J. 1983. Sexism, feminism and medicalism: A decade review of literature on gender and illness. *Sociology of Health and Illness* 5:62-82.

Coles, R. 1971. *Children of crisis*, vol. 2, *Migrants, sharecroppers, mountaineers*. Boston: Little, Brown.

Davis, D.L. 1982. Medical misinformation: Communication between outport Newfoundland women and their physician. Paper presented at the meeting of the American Anthropological Association, Washington, D.C.

Davis, D.L. 1983. Woman the worrier: Confronting feminist and biomedical archetypes of stress. *Women's Studies* 10:135-46.

Dornbran, L. n.d.. Unpublished interviews.

Duffin, L. 1978. The conspicuous consumptive: Woman as invalid. In *The nineteenth century woman: Her cultural and physical world*, eds. S. Delamont and L. Duffin, 27-55. New York: Barnes & Noble.

Eller, R. 1982. Harry Caudill and the burden of mountain liberalism. In *Critical essays in Appalachian life and culture*, eds. G. Edwards, R. Eller and J. Moser, Proceedings of the Fifth Annual Appalachian Studies Conference. Boone, N.C.: Appalachian Consortium Press.

Ehrenreich, B., and D. English. 1973. *Complaints and disorders: The sexual politics of sickness*. Glass Mountain Pamphlet No. 2. New York: Feminist Press.

Ehrenreich, B., and D. English. 1978. *For her own good: 150 years of the experts' advice to women*. New York: Anchor Press.

Fabrega. H. 1970. On the specificity of folk illnesses. *Southwestern Journal of Anthropology* 26:304-14.

Ferguson, K. 1984. *The feminist case against bureaucracy.* Philadelphia: Temple University Press.

Figlio, K. 1983. Chlorosis and chronic disease in nineteenth-century Britain: The social constitution of somatic illness in a capitalist society. In *Women and health: The politics of sex in medicine*, ed. E. Fee, 213-41. Farmingdale, N.Y.: Baywood Publishing Company.

Fisher, S.L. 1976. Victim-blaming in Appalachia. In *Appalachia: Social context past and present*, eds. B. Ergood and B. Kuhre, 139-48. Dubuque: Kendall/Hunt.

Flannery, M. 1982. Simple living and hard choices. *Hastings Center Report* 12:9-12.

Friedl, J. 1978. *Health care services and the Appalachian migrant.* Columbus: Ohio State University, Department of Anthropology.

Good, B.J., and M.J. Good. 1984. Toward a meaning centered analysis of popular illness categories: "Fright illness" and "heart disease" in Iran. In *Cultural conceptions of mental health and therapy*, eds. A.J. Marsella and G.M. White, 141-66. Dordecht: D. Reidel.

Harrison, P. 1982. Mothers in distress. *The Co-Evolution Quarterly* Winter:26-31.

Hechtlinger, A. 1970. *The great patent medicine era.* New York: Grosset and Dunlap.

Horton, C. 1984. Women have headaches, men have backaches: Patterns of illness in an Appalachian community. *Social Science and Medicine* 19:647-54.

Kleinman, A. 1980. *Patients and healers in the context of culture: An exploration of the borderland between anthropology, medicine, and psychiatry.* Berkeley: University of California Press.

Leighton, D.C., and N.C. Cline. 1968. The public health nurse as a mental health practitioner. In *Essays in medical anthropology*, ed. T. Weaver, 36-54. Athens: University of Georgia Press.

Lewis, H. 1976. Fatalism or the coal industry? In *Appalachia: Social context past and present*, eds. B. Ergood and B. Kuhre, 153-61. Dubuque: Kendall/Hunt.

Looff, D. 1971. *Appalachia's children.* Lexington: University Press of Kentucky.

Low, S. 1981. The meaning of *nervios*: A sociocultural analysis of symptom presentation in San Jose, Costa Rica. *Culture, Medicine and Psychiatry* 5:350-57.

Low, S. 1984. The biomedical response to *nervios.* Paper presented at the meeting of the American Anthropological Association, Denver.

Low, S., and K.R. Hammer. 1983. Nerves in Guatemala: An examination of cultural meanings. Paper presented at the meeting of the American Anthropological Association, Chicago.

Ludwig, A. 1982. "Nerves": A sociomedical diagnosis . . . of sorts. *American Journal of Psychotherapy* 26:350-57.

Ludwig, A., and B. Forrester. 1981. The condition of "nerves." *The Journal of the Kentucky Medical Association* 79:333-36.

Ludwig, A., and R. Forrester. 1982. Nerves, but not mentally. *Journal of Clinical Psychiatry* 43:187-90.

Mabry, J.J. 1964. Lay concepts of etiology. *Journal of Chronic Disease* 17:371-86.

Reissman, C.K. 1983. Women and medicalization: A new perspective. *Social Policy* 14:3-18.

Smith-Rosenberg, C., and C. Rosenberg. 1984. The female animal: Medical and biological views of woman and her role in nineteenth-century America. In *Women and health in America*, ed. J. W. Leavitt, 12-27. Madison: University of Wisconsin Press.

Thomas, S. 1983. Nostrum advertising and the image of woman as invalid in late Victorian America. *Journal of American Culture* 5:104-12.

Van Schaik, E. 1983. "My nerves bothers me but that's not all:" The meaning of nerves in eastern Kentucky. Masters diss., University of Kentucky, Lexington.

Walls, D.S. 1976. Central Appalachia: A peripheral region within an advanced capitalist society. *Journal of Sociology and Social Welfare* 4:232-47.

Weller, J. 1965. *Yesterday's people.* Lexington: University Press of Kentucky.

Wiesel, C., and M. Arny. 1952. Psychiatric study of coal miners in Eastern Kentucky. *American Journal of Psychiatry* 108:617-24.

Wood, A.D. 1984. "The fashionable diseases": Women's complaints and their treatment in nineteenth-century America. In *Women and health in America,* ed. J.W. Leavitt, 222-38. Madison: University of Wisconsin Press.

7

Social Support Networks of Families with Handicapped Children

CARL J. DUNST, CAROL M. TRIVETTE, AND ARTHUR H. CROSS

This paper presents findings from a study examining the mediating effects of social support on the personal and familial well-being of parents of handicapped children. The study was conducted in rural western North Carolina, in an area that includes eight Appalachian and four non-Appalachian counties (Appalachian Regional Commission 1977; Ergood 1976).[1]

Social system theory (Bronfenbrenner 1977, 1979; Caplan 1976; Cochran and Brassard 1979; Holahan 1977; Mitchell and Trickett 1980) was used to generate predictions regarding the relationships between social support networks and well-being. Our main hypothesis was that availability of social support would be inversely related to physical and emotional distress and family disintegration. There is a considerable body of evidence to indicate that the birth and rearing of a handicapped child can be an extremely devastating event for parents (e.g., Farber 1960; Gath 1977; Olshansky 1962; Schonell and Watts 1956; Stanko 1973), but that social support can buffer or alleviate the emotional anguish of the parents and other family members (Gabel, McDowell, and Cerreto 1983; McCubbin et al. 1980; Mitchell and Trickett 1980).

Social networks have long been viewed as powerful sources of social support. Bott (1971) defined social networks as "all or some of the social units (individuals or groups) with whom an individual is in contact" (p. 320). There is nearly unanimous agreement among social network theorists that social support networks function to nurture and sustain links among persons who are supportive of one another on a day-to-day basis and in times of need and crises. Broadly defined, social support includes emotional, psychological, physical, and monetary assistance that lessens or alleviates stresses associated with different life events (Cohen and Syme 1985).

Operationally, one can distinguish between *informal* and *formal* support networks. Informal social support networks include both individuals (kin, friends, neighbors, minister, etc.) and social groups (e.g., church) accessible to provide support to a target person as part of daily life. Formal support networks include both professionals (physicians, psychologists, social workers, etc.) and agencies (mental health centers, early intervention programs, etc.) formally organized, on an a priori basis, to provide support services to persons seeking help or assistance (Mitchell and Trickett 1980).

Gourash (1978) delineated four ways informal social networks influence decisions about seeking help. These include "(a) buffering the experience of stress which obviates the need for [professional] help, (b) precluding the necessity for professional assistance through the provision of instrumental and affective support, (c) acting as a screening and referral agent to professional services, and (d) transmitting attitudes, values, and norms about help-seeking" (p. 516). Available evidence from the mental health field (e.g., Mitchell and Trickett 1980) suggests that influences (a) and (b) are oftentimes sufficient in alleviating the need for professional services in dealing with most day-to-day crises and stresses. Influences (c) and (d) come into play whenever needed information or support cannot be provided by one's personal informal social network (Granovetter 1973). Implicit in Gourash's (1978) help-seeking model is the hypothesis that the stronger and more dominant informal social support networks are, the lower the probability will be that help is sought from formal social support systems.

Social systems theory seems especially useful for studying mental-health related problems in Appalachia. First, there is some evidence that there is a higher prevalence of mental illness and associated emotional problems among individuals residing in Appalachia (Finney 1969; Lee, Gianturco, and Eisdorfer 1974; Swift, Decker, and McKeown 1975). Second, there is evidence to indicate that Appalachians seek professional help for emotional problems less frequently than do non-Appalachians (Keefe, Chapter 8; Lee et al. 1974). Third, it is generally the case that informal social support network members, particularly nuclear and extended family, are often times the primary sources of assistance and help in dealing with personal emotional problems in Appalachia (Keefe, Chapter 2; Looff 1973). Keefe (Chapter 2) notes that the Appalachian family can be an extremely strong source of "stability, security, and other important psychological benefits" for dealing with emotional problems. This particular set of conditions raises two important questions: first, do Appalachian families differ from non-Appalachian families with regard to their sources of social support? and second, if so, are the differential types of support sufficient in buffering and lessening emotional problems?

SOCIAL SUPPORT AND THE APPALACHIAN FAMILY

Batteau (1979/80) noted that the Appalachian family structurally is composed of relationships based on both inclusion (kinship) and reciprocity (neighborliness). At the turn of the century, Vincent (1898) made note of the fact that the social organization of the Appalachian family unit was based upon kinship. Brown and Schwarzweller's (1971) analysis of the Appalachian family led them to conclude that the family system is based upon both conjugal and extended family relationships where the latter performs such vital functions as assuring well-being in times of need and crises. The Appalachian family traditionally has been characterized as self-reliant and strongly dependent upon informal social support structures for managing life crises and coping with hardships (Batteau 1979/80; Brown and Schwarzweller 1971; Jones 1976; Lewis, Kobak, and Johnson 1978).

The view of the Appalachian family as part of an informal social support network that mediates well-being and coping provides tentative evidence concerning why Appalachians seek professional help for emotional problems less frequently than non-Appalachians. It may be that the personal social networks of emotionally distressed individuals are sufficient enough to buffer and alleviate most day-to-day stresses. This contention seems most tenable in situations where the particular stress-producing life events are ones that network members have experienced themselves (either directly and indirectly) and thus are likely to be able to offer assistance, advice, and so on to lessen the emotional reactions to the stressful events. However, there are instances where certain life events are of infrequent occurrence, and consequently network members are less likely to be able to offer advice or provide help that alleviates emotional distress. The birth and rearing of a handicapped child is an unfortunate but nonetheless potentially revealing life event that can shed light on the relationships between support, culture, and emotional disturbances.

There is evidence to indicate that families of handicapped children have less informal social support available to them than families of normally developing children (Friedrich and Friedrich 1981; McAllister, Butler, and Lei 1973; McDowell and Gabel 1979;). In terms of Gourash's (1978) help-seeking model described earlier, one would hypothesize that because less social support is available to families of handicapped children, informal support networks are less likely to buffer the stresses and demands of the birth and rearing of the child. Moreover, because extended family members and members of the parents' kinship units are less likely to be knowledgeable about handicapping conditions (Gabel 1979), one would expect that the likelihood of seeking help from a formal social support network would be increased considerably. If the view of the Appalachian family as self-reliant and less dependent upon formal support networks is at all accurate, however, then one would expect these families to find such extrafamily support networks less helpful with regard to rearing their handicapped child. In addition, because Appalachian families would seek outside help less often and because informal social support networks would not be expected to buffer the stresses of rearing a handicapped child, it would be expected that one would find elevated levels of stress-related problems in Appalachian families with handicapped children.

RESEARCH QUESTIONS AND METHODOLOGY

The findings presented here are from a larger investigation examining the relationships among different types of social support and (1) parental emotional and physical well-being, (2) family integrity, (3) parental expectations for their handicapped child, and (4) child behavioral and developmental characteristics (see Dunst and Trivette 1984; Dunst, Trivette, and Cross 1986a, 1986b; Trivette and Dunst 1987). Two major research questions were asked as part of the analyses for the present report:

1. Do Appalachian and non-Appalachian families differ in terms of availability and satisfaction with sources of support from informal and formal social network members? The analyses performed to answer this question use Hollingshead's (1975) measure of Social Economic Status (SES) as an independent variable to test for interactions between SES and group membership (Appalachian vs. non-Appalachian).

2. Does number and quality of social support mediate personal and familial well-being? The analyses performed to answer this question included both SES and group membership (Appalachian vs. non-

Table 7.1. Selected Characteristics of the Sample Families

Characteristics	Mean	SD	Range
Parents			
Mother's age (years)	28.98	8.52	13-58
Father's age (years)	33.17	8.09	21-61
Mother's educational level[a]	11.50	2.57	3-18
Father's educational level[a]	11.53	2.76	6-20
Social economic status[b]	26.96	12.88	8-61
Gross monthly income (dollars)	1173.90	743.73	127-4000
Children			
Chronological age (months)	37.52	13.75	8-78
Mental age (months)	22.90	12.70	1-65
Intelligence quotient	63.88	26.10	10-115
Social-adaptive age (months)	24.75	13.00	1-60
Social quotient	70.70	27.98	10-125

[a]Highest grade completed.
[b]Hollingshead (1975) five-level model.

Appalachian) as independent variables to test for interactions between the three major measures.

    The subjects were 131 parents (89 mothers and 42 fathers) of handicapped children enrolled in the Family, Infant and Preschool Program.[2] Eighty-five percent of the parents in the sample were married, while the remaining 15 percent were single, widowed, separated, or divorced. The percentage of single-parent households is nearly identical to that in the general southern Appalachian region (Appalachian Regional Commission 1978).

    Selected characteristics of the families are presented in Table 7.1. On the average, both the mothers and fathers were about thirty years of age and both parents completed just less than twelve years of school. In terms of Hollingshead's (1975) five-level model of SES, the sample, on the average, fell into the second lowest social strata. It is especially noteworthy that 44 percent of the sample fell within the lowest social strata, indicating that the entire parent population was generally of low SES. Table 7.1 shows considerable variability with regard to gross monthly income, indicating that the families were quite heterogeneous in their financial status. Nearly half (48%) of the sample had average gross yearly incomes of under $12,000, however.

Table 7.1 shows that the children, on the average, were about three years of age and manifested a fifteen-month delay in their development. Their level of mental performance placed the group as a whole in the mild range of mental retardation (Grossman 1973), although the sample varied from profound to not retarded. The diagnoses of the children's handicaps included cerebral palsy (24 percent), chromosomal abberations (6 percent), cranial anomalies and spina bifida (12 percent), mental retardation due to unknown causes (23 percent), language impairment (18 percent), and developmental risk due to environmental factors (17 percent). Fifty-seven percent of the children were boys and 43 percent girls.

The parents completed a number of questionnaires as part of their participation in this study, including the Family Support Scale (Dunst, Jenkins, and Trivette 1984) and the Questionnaire on Resources and Stress (Holroyd 1974). Both scales are based on self-reports. Over 90 percent of the parents were able to read well enough to complete the quesionnaires independently. The remaining parents had the scales read to them by a relative, a friend, or a staff member of the Family, Infant and Preschool Program who worked with the family.

The Family Support Scale is designed to measure how helpful different sources of support have been to parents in terms of the care of their preschool-aged child. For eighteen potential sources of support, parents indicate the extent to which each was helpful to them during the six-month period immediately preceding completion of the scale. Ratings are made on a five-point Likert scale ranging from Not At all Helpful (zero) to Extremely Helpful (4). The sources of support on the scale includes items that assess the availability and satisfaction (helpfulness) of support from both informal (eleven items) and formal (seven items) support networks.

The Family Support Scale (FSS) has been shown to have excellent psychometric properties (Dunst, Jenkins, and Trivette 1984). Test-retest reliability estimates taken one month apart yielded an average r of .75 (SD = .17) for the separate scale items and a $r = .91$ for the total scale scores. The split-half reliability of the scale adjusted for length was $r = .75$. Factor analysis of the scale yielded six separate orthogonal factors indicating that the FSS is measuring independent sources of support.

The Questionnaire on Resources and Stress (QRS) is a true-false questionnaire designed to assess a number of dimensions of stress, well-being, and family integrity as they relate to the care of a handicapped child.[3] Two separate sets of scales on the QRS were included as part of analyses reported here: personal problems of the respondent as related to their handicapped child (6 scales);[4] and family problems related to the handicapped child (3 scales). The six personal-problems scales assess (1) poor health or mood of the respondent, (2) time demands placed upon the respondent by the handicapped child, (3) negative attitudes of the respondent toward his or her handicapped child, (4) dependency of the child on the respondent, (5) overcommitment of care for the child by the respondent, and (6) the respondent's degree of pessimism in terms of the future status of the child. The three family scales assess (1) lack of family integration, (2) limits placed on family opportunities due to the child's handicap, and (3) financial problems and burdens placed on the family by the child's handicap.

The question of whether Appalachian families differed from non-Appalachian families in terms of social support available to them was answered through a series of Group Membership (Appalachian vs. non-Appalachian) × SES (low vs. high) analyses of variance.[5] The Low SES group included all families who fell within the lowest social strata according to Hollingshead's (1975) five-level model, and the High SES group included all families who fell in levels two through five. This grouping schema results, respectively, in 44 percent and 56 percent of the sample falling into the two SES groups.

A series of Groups (Appalachian vs. non-Appalachian) × SES (low vs. high) × Social Support (low vs. high) analyses of covariance were used to answer the question whether social support mediated personal and familial well-being. Analyses were performed separately for the *number* of support networks and the *qualitative ratings* of social support. Median splits of both the number of social supports networks available to the respondent and the social support scores (sum of the ratings of the 18 FSS sources of support) were used for grouping the subjects as having low or high support. The covariates were the child's level of retardation as measured by Mental Development Index (MDI) scores (Bayley 1969), or Stanford-Binet Intelligence Quotient (IQ) scores (Terman & Merrill 1960) and the child's chronological age.

Main effects were tested at the .10 level of significance and interaction effects tested at the .05 level of significance.

RESULTS

Table 7.2 presents the mean scores on the FSS. Eight comparisons between the Appalachian and non-Appalachian groups were statis-

Table 7.2. Mean Support Scores on the Family Support Scale

Social Support Measures	Group				SES			
	Appalachian (N=94)	Non-Appalachian (N=37)	F(1127)	p	Low (N=58)	High (N=73)	F(1127)	p
Overall Indexes								
Number of sources of support	11.19	12.37	3.48	< .06	11.44	11.59	.20	ns
Total support scales	28.63	32.59	2.66	ns	28.69	30.59	.20	ns
Informal support network scores[a]	16.09	18.59	1.53	ns	15.41	17.90	1.49	ns
Formal support network scores	12.53	14.11	2.71	< .10	13.28	12.73	.66	ns
Scale Items								
Respondent's parents	2.31	2.06	.54	ns	2.36	2.14	.21	ns
Spouse's[b] parents	1.76	1.83	.04	ns	1.45	2.04	3.30	< .07
Respondent's relatives/kin	1.44	1.32	.19	ns	1.53	1.31	.27	ns
Spouse's relatives/kin	1.18	1.33	.10	ns	1.05	1.35	3.57	< .07
Spouse	2.88	3.16	.01	ns	2.26	3.51	19.50	< .001
Friends	1.36	1.89	4.23	< .05	1.53	1.49	.34	ns
Spouse's friends	.99	1.52	3.85	< .05	.93	1.31	.66	ns
Respondent's children	1.40	1.48	.05	ns	1.46	1.39	.02	ns
Other parents	.75	1.11	2.14	ns	.81	.89	.00	ns

Table 7.2, *continued*

Social Support Measures	Group				SES			
	Appalachian (N=94)	Non-Appalachian (N=37)	F(1127)	p	Low (N=58)	High (N=73)	F(1127)	p
Social groups/clubs	.26	.76	4.59	< .03	.33	.46	.32	ns
Church	1.75	2.14	3.34	< .07	1.69	1.99	.21	ns
Professional helpers	2.70	3.19	1.89	ns	2.78	2.89	.58	ns
Family/child's physician	2.34	2.81	3.02	< .09	2.33	2.58	.22	ns
Coworkers	.73	.84	.13	ns	.79	.74	.01	ns
Parent support group	.85	.54	.73	ns	.69	.82	.01	ns
School/day-care center	1.65	1.92	.78	ns	1.79	1.67	.32	ns
Professional agencies	1.28	1.59	5.74	< .02	1.89	.96	16.59	< .001
Specialized early intervention services[c]	2.96	3.22	.01	ns	3.00	3.07	1.27	ns

[a]Informal support network scores were the sum of the ratings for the first eleven FSS scale items and the formal support network scores were the sum of the last seven FSS scale items.

[b]For single-parent respondents, the word *spouse* was replaced with *child's father* or *child's mother*.

[c]The item included the name of the program (Family, Infant and Preschool Program) that provided specialized services to the child and family.

Table 7.3. Mean Scale Scores on the Questionnaire on Resources and Stress.

Scales	Support[a]				Group				SES			
	Low (N=65)	High (N=65)	F (1120)	p	Appalachian (N=93)	Non-Appalachian (N=37)	F (1120)	p	Low (N=56)	High (N=74)	F (1120)	p
Personal Problems												
Poor health or mood (11)[b]	4.32	2.95	4.29	< .04	3.81	3.20	.34	ns	4.09	3.29	2.73	< .10
Excess time demands (14)	6.00	4.92	12.73	< .001	5.37	5.68	1.71	ns	5.51	5.41	.46	ns
Negative attitude (23)	7.74	7.29	2.85	< .10	7.65	7.23	.75	ns	7.39	7.62	.14	ns
Overprotection (13)	5.14	4.36	3.75	< .06	4.73	4.81	1.19	ns	4.82	4.70	.13	ns
Overcommitment (8)	4.26	3.00	.25	ns	3.07	3.11	.72	ns	3.10	3.07	.74	ns
Pessimism (13)	1.63	1.45	1.96	ns	1.43	1.84	3.14	< .08	1.59	1.51	.50	ns
Family Problems												
Family integration (23)	2.51	2.48	.30	ns	2.49	2.53	2.75	< .10	3.21	1.96	15.23	< .001
Family opportunities (9)	1.07	1.08	2.20	ns	1.13	.92	.60	ns	1.22	.96	.45	ns
Financial problems (17)	6.05	4.96	2.19	ns	5.89	4.53	.16	ns	7.67	3.86	27.53	< .001

Note: Higher QRS scores indicate more problems or stress.
[a]Median split of number of social support networks available to the respondent.
[b]The numbers in parentheses indicate the number of items on each QRS Scale.

tically significant: number of sources of support, formal support network scores, friends, spouse's friends, social groups/clubs, church, family or child's physician, and professional agencies. All analyses indicated that the non-Appalachian families found their social support systems more helpful in terms of the care of their handicapped child compared to the Appalachian families. It is noteworthy that 19 of the 22 comparisons favored the non-Appalachian families in terms of satisfaction with their social support networks, both informal and formal.

The comparisons between the low- and high-SES groups yielded statistically significant differences on four support measures: spouse's parents, spouse's relatives and kin, spouse, and professional agencies. These results showed that the low-SES respondents found their spouses and in-laws less helpful than did the high-SES group; and that the low-SES group found professional agencies (public health, social services, mental health, etc.) more helpful than did the high-SES respondents.

The series of ANOVAs (analysis of variation) yielded only two interactions between group membership and SES: church, F $(1127) = 4.79$, $p < .03$, and specialized early intervention services for the child and family, F $(1127) = 3.90$, $p < .05$. The interaction in which the church is a source of support revealed that the low-SES non-Appalachian families (M = 2.78) found the church more helpful than the low-SES Appalachian families (M = 1.49). The high-SES Appalachian (M = 2.04) and non-Appalachian (M = 1.93) families found the church equally helpful. The findings for the interaction involving the specialized early intervention services variable showed that the non-Appalachian high-SES group (M = 3.43) found this source of support more helpful than did the non-Appalachian low-SES group (M = 2.56). The two Appalachian groups found the source equally helpful (M = 2.84 and M = 3.08, respectively, for the high- and low-SES groups).

The QRS findings on the number of support sources are shown in Table 7.3. Four findings were statistically significant between the low- and high-support groups, on four of the six personal respondent scales: poor health or mood, excess time demands, negative attitude, and overprotection. The findings for the poor health or mood scale indicated that persons with larger social support networks reported fewer physical and emotional problems compared to the low-support group. The findings for the excess time demands scale indicated that persons with larger social support networks had fewer time demands placed upon them in terms of the day-to-day care of their handicapped

children. The high-support group also indicated having a more positive attitude toward their handicapped child. Respondents with
smaller social networks were the same individuals who reported being
more overprotective of their children. Taken together, these findings
suggest that the *size* of the respondents' social support network mediated the psychological adaptation and coping of the parents. Size
of network did not significantly relate to any of the family problem
scales.

There were only two significant differences between the Appalachian and non-Appalachian groups for all the QRS comparisons: pessimism, and family integration. These two significant findings
indicated that Appalachian families are somewhat more optimistic
about their children's future developmental status, and that their
families functioned as more integrated units despite the child's handicap.

Social economic status was found to be significantly related to three
QRS scales: poor health or mood, family integration, and financial
problems. Low-SES respondents reported having (1) more physical
and emotional problems, (2) less integrated family units, and (3) more
financial problems. The latter finding certainly was not unexpected.
The findings regarding the relationships between SES and personal
and familial well-being suggest that SES represents a type of personal
support that includes both economic and educational components
(Hollingshead 1975), and that this type of support in fact mediates
well-being as well as family integrity.

The series of nine ANOVAs yielded significant two-way interactions for three QRS scales: excess time demands, negative attitude,
and family opportunities. Only the interactions involving the time
demands scale qualified the main effects reported in Table 7.3.

The analysis for the excess time demands scale yielded significant
SES × Support, $F(1120) = 4.70$, $p < .04$; SES × Groups, $F(1120) = 5.73$,
$p < .02$; and Support × Groups, $F(1120) = 5.97$, $p < .02$, interactions.
The SES × Group interaction showed that the non-Appalachian low-
SES group ($M = 6.71$) reported having more time demands placed
upon them than the non-Appalachian high-SES group ($M = 5.35$). The
low-SES ($M = 5.28$) and high-SES ($M = 5.46$) Appalachian groups did
not differ. The Support × SES interaction revealed that the low-support low-SES group ($M = 6.25$) reported having more time demands
than the high-support low-SES group ($M = 4.66$). The high-SES low-
support ($M = 5.78$) and high-support ($M = 5.22$) groups did not differ.
The Support × Groups interaction indicated that the low-Support

non-Appalachian group (M = 7.22) reported having more time demands than the high-support non-Appalachian group (M = 4.85). The low-support (M = 5.69) and high-support (M = 4.97) Appalachian groups did not differ. Taken together, these interactions indicate the Appalachian families, regardless of SES or level of support, reported having fewer time demands. These findings indicated that Appalachian families who were low-SES or had minimal support were not adversely affected in terms of the amount of time demands placed upon them, whereas the non-Appalachian low-SES and low-support groups were.

A significant SES × Groups, F (1120) = 4.86, p<.03, interaction for the negative attitude scale indicated that the high-SES non-Appalachian group (M = 5.84) had a significantly more positive attitude toward their child than the low-SES non-Appalachian group (M = 8.44). Both the low-SES (M = 7.19) and the high-SES (M = 8.06) Appalachian groups had QRS scores comparable to the low-SES non-Appalachian group. These findings showed that SES differentially affected the attitude of the non-Appalachian but not the Appalachian groups.

A significant Support × Groups, F (1120) = 4.80, p<.03, interaction for the family opportunities scale revealed that the high-support non-Appalachian group (M = .70) had fewer limits placed upon their family compared to the low-support non-Appalachian group (M = 1.34). The two Appalachian groups—low-support (M = 1.00) and high-support (M = 1.29)—had family opportunities scores equal to that of the low-support non-Appalachian group. These findings indicated that social support differentially affected limits on family opportunities for the non-Appalachian but not the Appalachian groups.

Table 7.4 presents the findings on the social support scores of the QRS for the low- and high-support groups. Without exception, the mean scores for groups were in the predicted direction. There were statistically significant differences between the low- and high-support groups on five of the QRS scales: poor health or mood, excess time demands, overprotection, family integration, and family opportunities. The findings for the personal respondent scales are nearly identical to those found for the size of social networks. Respondents who indicated being more satisfied with the help provided by their social networks were the same individuals who reported having (1) less physical and emotional problems, (2) fewer time demands placed upon them, and (3) being less overprotective of their children.

Respondents who reported having more supportive social networks also indicated that their families functioned as more integrated

Table 7.4. Mean Scale Scores on the Questionnaire on Resources and Stress for the Total Social Support Scores

	Support[a]			
Scales	Low (N = 67)	High (N = 63)	F (1120)	p
Personal Problems				
Poor health or mood	4.48	2.7	6.89	<.01
Excess time demands	5.53	4.56	10.62	<.01
Negative attitudes	7.73	6.94	1.10	ns
Overprotective	5.12	4.36	4.65	<.05
Overcommitment	3.17	2.98	.33	ns
Pessimism	1.67	1.42	1.22	ns
Family Problems				
Family integration	2.80	2.00	2.73	<.10
Family opportunities	1.31	.82	3.44	<.07
Financial problems	6.00	4.98	1.83	ns

Note: The main effects for Groups and SES are identical to those reported in Table 7.3 and therefore are not repeated here.
[a]Median split of the total of the ratings for the 18 family support scale items.

units, where both the care of the handicapped child was shared among family members and the handicapped child did not place undue burdens upon the family. The significant findings between the low- and high-support groups on the limits on family opportunity scale indicated that persons with more supportive social networks were members of families where the child's handicap did not place limits on their family opportunities (e.g., going out to dinner). Together the findings regarding the relationship between support and family integrity indicate that the former in fact does mediate the latter.

None of the analyses yielded any significant interactions between the three main effects variables.

DISCUSSION

This study was designed to answer two major questions: (1) do Appalachian and non-Appalachian families differ in terms of their social support networks? and (2) does social support mediate personal and familial well-being with regard to the birth and rearing of a handicapped child? It was predicted that Appalachian and non-Appalachian families would differ in terms of the nature of their informal and formal social networks; that social support would mediate personal and familial well-being; and that Appalachianness would interact with social support in affecting well-being. Our discussion is divided into two sections corresponding to the two major research questions.

The results reported in this paper showed a trend for families from non-Appalachian counties to have more supportive social networks than families from Appalachian counties. More specifically, non-Appalachian families had significantly more sources of support available to them, and a number of sources were rated as more helpful in terms of the care of their handicapped child. In descending order, the individual sources of support rated by the respondents as more helpful were professional agencies, social groups and clubs, friends of the respondent, friends of the respondent's spouse, church, and the family or child's physician.

The findings regarding the differences in the support networks of Appalachian and non-Appalachian families provide partial support for the contention that Appalachian families are less dependent upon, or at least find more formal social support networks less helpful, than non-Appalachian families. The analyses showed that Appalachian families rated formal social support networks as being less supportive in terms of the care of their handicapped child. More specifically, Appalachian families rated professional agencies (social services, public health, mental health, etc.) and the family or child's primary health provider as less helpful compared to non-Appalachian familes. This particular finding is consistent with the popular characterization of the Appalachian family as self-reliant and less dependent upon formal sources of support (Batteau 1979/80; Brown and Schwarzweller 1971; Jones 1976; Lewis et al. 1978) and provides additional evidence to indicate that Appalachians rely less on professional help for dealing with emotional problems (Keefe, Chapter 2; Lee et al. 1974).

Contrary to expectations, the findings did not support the prediction that Appalachian families would indicate that informal social support networks were more helpful compared to non-Appalachian families. There were no significant findings to indicate that Appalachian and non-Appalachian families differed in terms of levels of support for any of the nuclear or extended family member FSS items. Significant differences were found on two nonkin informal support items (respondent's friends and spouse's friends), but these differences favored the non-Appalachian families. Of particular note is the finding that low-SES Appalachian families rated the church as being less helpful than low-SES non-Appalachian families. If the traditional view of the "poor" Appalachian family as strong churchgoers is accurate (Lewis et al. 1978), our findings would suggest that church attendance cannot be equated with church support.

The failure to find the predicted differences between the Appalachian and non-Appalachian families in terms of informal social support networks might be explained by the fact that, culturally, the two groups of parents were more alike than different to begin with. There is now general consensus that there is not *one* Appalachian culture but rather a series of cultures each with its own mores, values, beliefs, social rituals, etc. (Batteau 1979/80; Ergood & Kuhre 1976). For example, it is recognized that there are at least three major Appalachian subregions, which differ from one another in important cultural ways. Sociologically, proximal communities are more likely to be similar than distal communities, and the parents in the present study generally resided in adjacent counties. One could at least argue that the two groups of families included in this study were culturally alike and, as a result, can explain the lack of differences in terms of informal social support networks. However, two bits of data would argue against or at least qualify this explanation. First, the Appalachian and non-Appalachian families did differ on a number of support indexes. This would suggest that there are underlying differences between the groups, and these are perhaps, to a certain degree, cultural differences. Second, on several nuclear family social support items (see Table 7.2), there were differences between the two SES groups. This would indicate that SES rather than Appalachianness accounts for differences in informal social support networks.

As predicted, social support mediated both personal and familial well-being. Both the number of social support networks and the ratings of the helpfulness of support provided by network members was found to relate to (1) physical and emotional well-being, (2) time demands, and (3) overprotection of the handicapped child. Respondents with larger degrees of social support available reported (1) having fewer physical and emotional problems, (2) having fewer time demands in terms of the care of the handicapped child, and (3) being less protective of their child. Size of support network was also found to be related to attitudes toward the child, with the high-support group reporting a more positive attitude toward their children. Taken together, these results strongly indicate that the social support available to parents of handicapped children can buffer and lessen the stresses so often associated with the birth and rearing of a handi-capped child (Gabel et al. 1983). The findings also replicate those reported by our research group in a number of other studies (Dunst 1985; Dunst, Cooper, and Bolick, 1987; Dunst and Trivette 1984; Dunst, Trivette, et al. 1986a, 1986b; Dunst and Trivette in press; Dunst, Vance, and Cooper 1986).

It has generally been contended that a child's handicap and his or her intellectual impairment are *primary* stressors in these families (Beckman-Bell 1981). Our findings call this assertion into question. Of the seven significant differences found on the QRS personal re-spondent scales, six of the analyses showed that social support ac-counted for more of the variance than the two covariates (child IQ and age). Our findings indicate that social support is powerful enough to lessen the emotional reactions so often experienced by parents of handicapped children. Moreover, since neither Appalachianness nor SES were related to the personal problems of the respondents, it would appear further that social networks constitute potent sources of support that transcend both culture and economic or educational differences.

The results of our study showed that social support scores but not size of network, were significantly related to familial well-being. Both family integrity and family opportunities were affected by social sup-port. The families with larger degrees of support were the same fami-lies who were functioning as more integrated units and had less limits placed on them due to the child's handicap. On the family oppor-tunities scale, social support accounted for more of the variance than the covariates. On the family integration scale, however, both the covariates and SES accounted for more of the variance. This indicates that although social support was significantly related to family inte-gration, family disintegration correlates more with the child's intel-lectual impairment and the family's social economic status. These findings suggests complex relationship between social support, child, and economic or educational variables. Whereas personal well-being was primarily mediated by social support, familial well-being is ap-parently affected by a number of different mediating factors.

Although differences were found between the Appalachian and non-Appalachian groups in terms of availability and satisfaction (helpful-ness) with social support, the findings do not support the contention that lack of support adversely affected personal and familial well-being. The results also provide minimal support for the predicted interaction between Appalachianness and social support. Elevated levels of stress-related problems were found for the Appalachian group on only one QRS scale (family opportunities). For the only other Groups × Support interaction (excess time demands), level of stress-related problems were actually lower among the Appalachian respondents. These results indicate that despite having less social support available to them, what support Appalachian familes had was sufficient in buffering and lessening the emotional distress association with the rearing of their handicapped youngsters.

In summary, this study used social systems theory to examine the relationships between social support and well-being in Appalachian and non-Appalachian families with handicapped children. The general conclusion that can be made is that social support indeed can mediate well-being and lessen the distress typically associated with the rearing of a handicapped child. The mediating effects of social support were found to transcend cultural, economic, and educational differences. Moreover, and perhaps more important, social support generally accounted for more of the variance in terms of levels of emotional problems than did child's level of intellectual retardation. This finding strongly suggests that social support can be used as an intervention to lessen or even alleviate the distress associated with the birth and rearing of a handicapped child.

NOTES

The search reported in this chapter was supported, in part, by grants to the first author from the National Institute of Mental Health (MH38862) and the Research Section, Division of Mental Health, Mental Retardation, and Substance Abuse, North Carolina Department of Human Resources (#83527). Appreciation is extended to Pat Condrey and Norma Hunter for assistance in preparation of the manuscript.

1. The Appalachian counties included Alexander, Burke, Caldwell, McDowell, Mitchell, Rutherford, Wilkes, and Yancey. The non-Appalachian counties included Catawba, Cleveland, Iredell, and Rowan. For purposes of this paper, Appalachianness was defined by current county of residence and not birthplace. Because of potential biases resulting from this definition, Hollingshead's (1975) Social Economic Status (SES) was used to subdivide the sample into low- and high-SES groups. There are strong indicators that low SES families from rural areas are more likely to live their entire lives in the county in which they were born, and if they do migrate, relocations tend to be within the same county of residence (Schumaker and Stokols 1982; Sell and DeJong 1981; Speare, Kobrin, and Kingkade 1982). Consequently, it is reasonable to assume that at least for the low-SES Appalachian and non-Appalachian families, there is a high probability that current county of residence is the birthplace of the families as well as their ancestors.

2. The Family, Infant and Preschool Program (FIPP) is an outreach unit of Western Carolina Center, a regional facility serving handicapped persons in western North

Carolina. FIPP provides home-, center-, and community-based services to families of handicapped preschoolers in a 20-county area (see Dunst 1982, for a detailed description of the program).

3. The QRS also includes five child-problem scales, but these were not analyzed for this report since they did not relate to the two main research questions.

4. A seventh scale, Lack of Social Support, was not included since it did not provide information different from the Family Support Scale.

5. Subsequent multiple regression analysis of the data yielded nearly identical findings. Thus, although dichotomizing continuous variables as was done here generally is not recommended (Cohen and Cohen 1983), the ease of communication of ANOVA (analysis of variation) findings over those obtained by regression analysis was the reason for performing this type of analysis.

REFERENCES

Appalachian Regional Commission. 1977. *Appalachia: A reference book*. Washington, D.C.: Appalachian Regional Commission.

Appalachian Regional Commission. 1978. Appalachian children and their families: A statistical profile. Paper prepared for the conference on Raising a New Generation in Appalachia, Asheville, N.C.

Batteau, A. 1979/80. Appalachia and the concept of culture. *Appalachian Journal* 7:9-31.

Bayley, N. 1969. *The Bayley scales of infant development*. New York: Psychological Corporation.

Beckman-Bell, P. 1981. Child-related stress in families of handicapped children. *Topics in Early Childhood Special Education* 1(3):45-54.

Bott, E. 1971. *Family and social networks*. London: Tavistock Publications.

Bronfenbrenner, U. 1977. Toward an experimental ecology of human development. *American Psychologist* 32:513-31.

Bronfenbrenner, U. 1979. *The ecology of human development: Experiments by nature and design*. Cambridge: Harvard University Press.

Brown, J., and H. Schwarzweller. 1971. The Appalachian family. In *Change in rural Appalachia*, eds. J. Photiadis & H. Schwarzweller. Philadelphia: University of Pennsylvania Press.

Caplan, G. 1976. The family as support system. In *Support systems and mutual help*, eds. G. Caplan and M. Killilea. New York: Grune & Stratton.

Cochran, M., and J. Brassard. 1979. Child development and personal social networks. *Child Development* 50:601-16.

Cohen, J., and P. Cohen. 1983. *Applied multiple regression/ correlation analysis for the behavioral sciences*. 2nd ed. Hillsdale, N.J.: Erlbaum.

Cohen, S., and S.L. Syme. 1985. *Social support and health*. New York: Academic Press.

Dunst, C.J. 1982. Social support, early intervention, and institutional avoidance. Paper presented at the annual meeting of the Southeastern Association on Mental Deficiency, Louisville, Ky.

Dunst, C.J. 1985. Rethinking early intervention. *Analysis and Invervention in Developmental Disabilities* 5:165-201.

Dunst, C.J., C.S. Cooper, and F.A. Bolick. 1987. Supporting families of handicapped children. In *Special children, special risks: The maltreatment of children with disabilities*, eds. J. Barbarino, P.E. Brookhouser, and K. Authier, 17-46. New York: Aldine.

Dunst, C.J., V. Jenkins, and C.M. Trivette. 1984. The family support scale: Reliability and validity. *Wellness Perspectives* 1(4):45-52.

Dunst, C.J., and C.M. Trivette. 1984. Differential influences of social support on mentally retarded children and their families. Paper presented at the annual meeting of the American Psychological Association, Toronto.

Dunst, C.J., C.M. Trivette, and A.H. Cross. 1986a. Mediating influences of social support: Personal, family, and child outcomes. *American Journal of Mental Deficiency* 90:403-17.

Dunst, C.J., C.M. Trivette, and A.H. Cross. 1986b. Roles and support networks of mothers of handicapped children. In *Families of handicapped children: Needs and support across the lifespan*, eds. R. Fewell & P. Vadasy, 167-92. Austin, Tex.: PRO-ED.

Dunst, C.J., and C.M. Trivette. In press. Toward experimental evaluation of the Family, Infant and Preschool Program. In *Evaluating Family Programs*, eds. H. Weiss and F. Jacobs. New York: Aldine.

Dunst, C.J., S.D. Vance, and C.S. Cooper. 1986. A social systems perspective of adolescent pregnancy: Determinants of parent and parent-child behavior. *Infant Mental Health Journal* 7:34-48.

Ergood, B. 1976. Toward a definition of Appalachia. In *Appalachia: Social context past and present*, eds. B. Ergood & B. Kuhre. Dubuque: Kendall/Hunt.

Ergood, B., and B. Kuhre, eds. 1976. *Appalachia: Social context past and present*. Dubuque: Kendall/Hunt.

Farber, B. 1960. Family organization and crisis: Maintenance of integration in families with a severely mentally retarded child. Serial No. 7. *Monographs of the Society for Child Development* 25:1.

Finney, J., ed. 1969. *Cultural change, mental health, and poverty*. Lexington: University Press of Kentucky.

Friedrich, W., and W. Friedrich. 1981. Psychosocial assets of parents of handicapped and nonhandicapped children. *American Journal of Mental Deficiency* 85:551-53.

Gabel, H. 1979. The Family, infant and toddler project: Early intervention for rural families of retarded children. In *MR/DD rural services . . . it is time*, ed. R. Schalock. Washington, D.C.: Institute for Comprehensive Planning.

Gabel, H., J. McDowell, and M. Cerreto. 1983. Family adaptation to the handicapped infant. In *Educating handicapped infants*, eds. S.G. Garwood and R. Fewell. Rockville, Md.: Aspen.

Gath, A. 1977. The impact of an abnormal child upon the parents. *British Journal of Psychiatry* 130:405-10.

Gourash, N. 1978. Help seeking: A review of the literature. *American Journal of Community Psychology* 6:499-517.

Granovetter, M. 1973. The strength of weak ties. *American Journal of Sociology* 78:13-60.

Grossman, H., ed. 1973. *Manual on terminology and classification in mental retardation*. Washington, D.C.: American Association on Mental Deficiency.

Holahan, C.J. 1977. Social ecology. In *Community psychology in transition*, eds. I. Iscap, B. Bloom, and C. Spielberger. New York: Wiley.

Hollingshead, A.B. 1975. Four factor index of social status. Unpublished paper, Department of Sociology, Yale University, New Haven.

Holroyd, J. 1974. The questionnaire on resources and stress: An instrument to measure family responses to a handicapped child. *Journal of Community Psychology* 2:92-94.

Jones, L. 1976. Appalachian values. In *Appalachia: Social context past and present*, eds. B. Ergood and B. Kuhre. Dubuque: Kendall/Hunt.

Lee, S., D. Gianturco, and C. Eisdorfer. 1974. Community mental health center accessibility: A survey of the rural poor. *Archives of General Psychiatry* 31:335-39.

Lewis, H., S. Kobak, and L. Johnson. 1978. Family, religion and colonialism in central Appalachia. In *Colonialism in modern America: The Appalachian case*, eds. H. Lewis, L. Johnson, and D. Askin. Boone, N.C.: Appalachian Consortium Press.

Looff, D. 1973. Rural Appalachians and their attitudes toward health. In *Rural and Appalachian health*, eds. R. Nolan and J. Schwartz. Springfield, Ill.: Charles C. Thomas.

McAllister, R., E. Butler, and T. Lei. 1973. Patterns of social interaction among families of behaviorally retarded children. *Journal of Marriage and the Family* 35:93-100.

McCubbin, H., C. Joy, A.E. Cauble, J. Comeau, J. Patterson, and R. Needle. 1980. Family stress and coping: A decade review. *Journal of Marriage and Family* 42:855-71.

McDowell, J., and H. Gabel. 1979. Social support among mothers of mentally retarded infants. Unpublished paper, George Peabody College of Vanderbilt University, Nashville.

Mitchell, R.E., and E.J. Trickett. 1980. Social networks as mediators of social support: An analysis of the effects and determinants of social networks. *Community Mental Health Journal* 16:27-43.

Olshansky, S. 1962. Chronic sorrow: A response to having a mentally defective child. *Social Casework* 43:191-94.

Schonell, R., and B. Watts. 1956. A first survey of the effects of a subnormal child on the family unit. *American Journal of Mental Deficiency* 61:201-19.

Schumaker, S., and D. Stokols. 1982. Residential mobility as a social issue and research topic. *Journal of Social Issues* 38:1-19.

Sell, R., and G. DeJong. 1981. Deciding whether to move: Mobility, wishful thinking and adjustment. *Sociology and Social Research* 67:146-65.

Speare, A., F. Korbrin, and W. Kingkade. 1982. The influence of socioeconomic bonds and satisfaction on interstate mobility. *Social Forces* 61:551-74.

Stanko, B. 1973. Crisis intervention after the birth of a defective child. *Canadian Nurse* 69:27.

Swift, B., R. Decker, and M. McKeown. 1975. Mental health in Appalachia: An emerging problem. *Appalachia* 9:36-44.

Terman, L., and M. Merrill. 1960. *Stanford-Binet Intelligence Scale*. Boston: Houghton-Mifflin.

Trivette, C.M., and C.J. Dunst. 1987. Proactive influences of social support in families of handicapped children. In *Family strengths. Pathways to Well-being*, vol. 8-9, eds. H.G. Lingren, L. Kimmons, P. Lee, G. Rowe, L. Rottman, L. Schwab, and R. Williams, 391-405. Lincoln: University of Nebraska Press.

Vincent, G. 1898. A retarded frontier. *American Journal of Sociology* 4:1-20.

PART III

Mental Health Service Utilization in the Mountains

8

Factors Affecting the Use of
Mental Health Services: A Review

SUSAN EMLEY KEEFE

Factors affecting mental health service utilization are diverse and complex. Investigation of these factors has received considerable attention, especially with regard to disadvantaged groups, including ethnic minorities, the poor, and rural residents (e.g., Barrera 1978; Garrison 1975; Kaplan and Roman 1973; Miller 1966). For Appalachians, however, few such studies exist. The purpose of this paper is to briefly review relevant factors affecting mountaineers' use of mental health services and to conclude with recommendations for the improvement of mental health service delivery.

One of the difficulties in reviewing what has been written about Appalachians and mental health is determining the extent to which generalizations can be made. Mountaineers are not a homogeneous population. Although Appalachians are primarily residents of rural areas, there are metropolitan centers in the region. Although a high proportion of mountaineers live in poverty, there are also local elites and a significant middle class. Although some mountain people still carry on a folk tradition, others have joined the mainstream. In many of the studies reviewed, little attempt has been made by authors to establish the extent to which traits are tied to specific subpopulations. Future research must be concerned more with distinctions within the region. What follows might best be offered as a compilation of hypotheses in need of testing rather than pronouncements about the Appalachian population.

For the purpose of this review, it is useful to distinguish two basic types of factors affecting mental health service utilization by Appalachians: cultural and institutional. Cultural factors are those that characterize the client and institutional factors are those that characterize mental health services. In other words, it is assumed that the use of mental health services is affected by the attitudes and way of life of Appalachian people *and* by the attitudes and organizational predispositions of mental health professionals.

CULTURAL FACTORS

Illness behavior, the way in which a person deals with pain and sickness, is shaped to a great extent by culture. In Appalachia, the response to illness in general is one of fear (Looff 1971; Weller 1965).
Researchers suggest that this is the result of a rural way of life, where
physical strength is essential. Illness is also a threat to family solidarity, which is highly valued in Appalachian society (Looff 1973). It
appears that some abnormal states are not identified by mountaineers
as true sickness, perhaps because they are not threatening in the
foregoing ways. Pearsall (1962), for example, found that colds, sore
throats, and asthma, among others, are not considered to be illnesses
but instead are accepted as part of the normal human condition. Appalachians tend to downplay illness, preferring to ignore and endure
many symptoms and to resort to self-doctoring rather than going to
a physician. Illness often becomes life-threatening before a physician
is consulted (Pearsall 1962). Researchers have labeled this attitude
fatalism or, more neutrally, stoicism in the face of illness (Friedl 1978;
Hochstrasser and Nickerson 1966; Pearsall 1962). It may stem from
the general fear of illness but it may also be due to lack of money,
lack of faith in orthodox medicine, and the difficulty in locating medical practitioners in a rural area.

Although little reference to illness behavior with regard to mental
illness is found in the literature, we can assume that it is also feared
and endured rather than treated in any standard way. In fact, Weller
finds "the whole subject of mental illness is simply foreign to mountain people" (1965, p. 119). There is evidence, however, that mental
illness is identified by mountaineers. One fairly common affliction is
called nerves (see Van Schaik, Chapter 6). Even though mental illness
is recognized and named in Appalachia, there appears to be little
acceptance of professional mental health care. Weller states that "the
psychiatrist's care can be accepted only if he is called a 'nerve doctor' "
(1965, p. 119). In a study of health needs in eastern Kentucky, Steinman (1970) found psychiatry among the most difficult referrals to
complete.

The perceived cause of mental illness may be one reason for the
failure to seek professional treatment. Numerous researchers find that
mountaineers often believe illness is the will of God or supernatural
punishment for sins (Friedl 1978; Herlihy 1963; Hochstrasser and
Nickerson 1966). There is also a traditional magical belief that a pregnant woman's behavior or experiences may result in "marking" the
unborn child (Stekert 1971; Stuart 1966). Although this applies pri-

marily to birthmarks, "marking" is also believed to affect the emotional disposition of the child (for example, "The child of a woman who is greatly frightened while pregnant will be of a nervous disposition" Hand 1961, #197). Pearsall (1962), moreover, observes among mountaineers a lack of understanding of or faith in "scientific" medicine; given this and the belief in supernatural causation, it is not surprising that mental health services often are not utilized.

Rather than seek professional mental health care, Appalachians typically turn to other sources of help with mental health problems. The primary source of support is the family (see Keefe, Chapter 2). Looff, for instance, speaks of "the traditional tendencies of the southern Appalachian individual to attempt to cope with anxiety by turning inward in his close family system" (1973, p. 8). Appalachia is a kin-based society and relatives are relied upon for advice and emotional support. Middle-class mainstream Americans also rely on the family, but it tends to be limited to the nuclear family, and friends are often just as important in providing emotional support (Keefe, Padilla, and Carlos 1979). In Appalachia, relatives beyond the nuclear family are significant helpers and the family is far more important to the individual than nonkin. Looff and Smith (1969) contend that this family intensiveness promotes certain types of emotional problems, such as school phobia and other dependency-related problems. But we can also assume the strong extended family provides stability, security, and other important psychological benefits.

There are additional sources of treatment that may be appealed to more commonly in Appalachia than elsewhere. Religion and faith healing are traditional alternatives to orthodox medical care. Appalachians belong primarily to fundamentalist, sectarian Protestant churches; Holiness and Pentecostal churches proliferate in addition to fundamentalist Baptist and Methodist congregations. Humphrey (1974) stresses the emotional quality of religion in the mountains, and Holt (1940) observes that religious involvement is an important means of handling stress among mountaineers. Time is taken during religious services to ask for supernatural help in healing the sick. Some healing services are more instrumental, including such acts as the laying on of hands to cast out devils among members of the snake-handling sect (Kane 1974). Individual prayer, of course, is also relied upon for help with health problems (Pearsall 1960, 1962). More specifically, certain Bible verses, such as Ezekiel 16, may be repeated to treat particular ailments or for general comfort (Hill 1976; Wigginton 1972).

Folk medicine is another alternative for treatment in times of stress.

The *Foxfire* volumes have popularized the home remedies of mountaineers. Folk treatments for somatic symptoms, such as insomnia and stomach upsets, as well as more specifically emotional distress including nightmares and personality disorders, are mentioned (see also Long 1962). Several authors state that folk medicine is especially common for treating minor ailments (Hochstrasser and Nickerson 1966; Pearsall 1962; Stekert 1971; Weller 1965). Steinman (1970), however, found only 5% of 2190 households surveyed in an eastern Kentucky county had blood tonics or home remedies for colds and stomach complaints. There is some reason to believe, then, that folk medicine is declining in importance; and its importance is likely to be greater among the elderly and the more isolated rural poor.

There are folk healers in Appalachia but the literature does not indicate that they are asked to treat emotional problems. Folk healers include "granny midwives" (Osgood, Hochstrasser, and Deuschle 1966) and local specialists with supernatural powers who treat "thrash" (thrush, an infant fungal infection of the mouth), draw the "fire" out of burns, stop bleeding, and remove warts (Friedl 1978; Stekert 1971; Wigginton 1972).

Orthodox health practitioners may be consulted for emotional problems, but chances are Appalachians will turn to a physician rather than a mental health professional. The fear and suspicion of doctors found by numerous researchers, however, is likely to limit their usefulness (Coles 1967; Friedl 1978; Looff 1971; Stekert 1971; Weller 1965). Stekert (1971) points out that Appalachians also consult marginal practitioners such as chiropractors, who specialize in treating body aches that may have an emotional etiology, and their techniques often incorporate the personal attention highly valued by mountain people. The value of personalism is one reason Appalachians fail to utilize agencies and clinics that are unfamiliar (Looff 1971). Appalachians, of course, may not only avoid professional mental health services but may simply be unaware of them, as they are of other health services (Friedl 1978).

In this brief review of cultural factors, it is important to reemphasize that many of these traits are probably only characteristic of certain segments of the population. Most studies in Appalachia have concentrated on the rural poor. It is likely that the belief in supernatural causation, reliance on folk medicine, and fear of doctors apply primarily to this subgroup. Other traits such as the reliance on the family and the desire for personalism may be found more generally. These relationships await substantiation through comparative research.

INSTITUTIONAL FACTORS

The same qualification needs to be made with respect to the institutional factors, many of which apply only to the rural poor in Appalachia. Furthermore, many of these factors are true not only for those in Appalachia but for the poor and rural dwellers in general in the United States.

One of the most obvious problems in the delivery of mental health services in Appalachia is accessibility. Unlike the vast majority of the U.S. population, Appalachians are primarily rural dwellers. The location of clinics in towns and cities requires that rural residents travel inconvenient distances to receive treatment. This may create impossible problems for families in which there is only one car or the wife does not drive, especially since public transportation is generally unavailable in rural areas.

Another problem in mental health service delivery in Appalachia concerns social class factors. Research on mental health treatment has confirmed the difficulties created when middle-class therapists treat low-income clients. In Appalachia, more than in the United States at large, a high proportion of the population has a low income. In 1983, 18% lived in poverty (compared to 14% nationally) and the average income was 85% of the national income. As a result, Appalachian mental health clinics might expect an extensive lower-class clientele. One of the difficulties in treating the poor concerns the middle-class therapist's training in and expectation for verbal therapy. The poor are generally less educated, less verbal, and more interested in instrumental intervention. Aware of the nonverbal character of many mountain people, Looff (1971, p. 139) cites the need for "action-oriented, crisis-model approaches" to therapy in Appalachia. In addition to the treatment of emotional problems, the poor may expect mental health professionals to deal with interrelated problems requiring immediate attention, such as unemployment or inadequate housing. Although these are usually considered beyond the purview of mental health practitioners, it may be impossible to attack the emotional problems until these basic life problems are solved. Intervention as a mediator or active participant in helping clients solve basic life problems involves a change in the therapist's traditional role, but it may be very successful in relieving the client's overall stress (Burruel and Chavez 1974). This new role is made easier in multiservice centers, which now are increasingly common. The middle-class orientation of mental health agency organization also affects utilization (Looff 1973).

The poor, for example, are generally less accustomed to a life regulated by the clock and the habit of making and keeping appointments.

Cultural conflicts are as significant as class conflicts in mental health service utilization. As reviewed previously, Appalachian people have their own cultural conception about the causes and symptoms of mental illness and the appropriate modes of treatment. These do not tend to match the concepts used by mental health practitioners, thus creating a gap in communication. A particular complex of Appalachian behavioral traits that Hicks (1976) calls the "ethic of neutrality" may pose further problems for communication between Appalachians and mainstream therapists (see also Beaver 1986). According to Hicks, the ethic consists of four restrictions:

1. One must mind one's own business.
2. One must not be assertive, aggressive, or call attention to oneself.
3. One must not assume authority over others (violating the presumption of equality).
4. One must avoid argument and seek agreement.

These directives, especially to mind one's own business and not assume authority, would appear to make therapeutic intervention difficult at best. In suggesting means of intervention to nurses working with mountaineers who observe the ethic of neutrality, Tripp-Reimer and Friedl (1977) advise the following:

1. Be directive but not coercive in assisting the client to find alternatives.
2. Approach sensitive topics with indirect questions and suggestions.
3. Recognize that the client may be very sensitive to perceived criticism.

More basic to problems in communication is the language barrier. Mountaineers have a distinct accent and use a variant of standard English that many times makes it difficult for others to understand what is being said (Snow 1976; Stekert 1971). Not only do cultural patterns affect the mode of communication, they also influence the content. Many suggestions that might be made by a non-Appalachian therapist can conflict with Appalachian concepts about child rearing, extended family ties, gender role definitions, and so on. Finally, there is a need to recognize that prejudice may influence mental health service delivery. In-migrant mental health practitioners may have intolerant attitudes toward mountaineers, who are negatively stereotyped as hillbillies. Researchers have observed that this is true many times of health care specialists in general (Rogers and Rogers 1971; Stekert 1971).

RECOMMENDATIONS

Having reviewed a number of cultural and institutional factors affecting mental health service utilization in Appalachia, we can conclude with some specific recommendations for improving the delivery of services.

1. Work to increase public awareness of mental health services. Mental health services must actively ensure that people are aware of the location of clinics and the types of services offered. Public education aimed particularly at the rural poor is needed. Working with local schools and churches would be most effective. This would also provide access to community networks where referrals might begin. As Looff (1973) suggests, mental health services need to actively seek out clients among the rural poor.

2. Locate mental health clinics for maximum accessibility. Considering the rural nature of Appalachia, mental health facilities should undertake substantial decentralization in order to reach clients. This might involve sending therapists into small communities on certain days of the week to meet local clients or setting up branch units outside central towns and cities. In urban areas, a single health services center incorporating mental health services would ensure greater public familiarity with the facility and might help to overcome the stigma of a "mental" health center.

3. Adopt flexible services to meet the needs of low-income people. Mental health services should allow some flexibility in clinic hours and appointment schedules so that therapists are available in the evenings and for crisis counseling. Therapies appropriate for nonverbal-oriented clients should be available.

4. Involve Appalachians in the mental health care system. The best way to ensure mental health services are culturally appropriate is to involve native Appalachians in the organization and delivery of services. Ideally, this would mean including therapists of Appalachian descent. Appalachian paraprofessionals, however, can also be important adjuncts in providing mental health care. Several researchers note the benefits of using health care personnel who are familiar with the local way of life and the families in need as well as being known

and trusted by the people (Hochstrasser and Nickerson 1966; Looff 1971; Pearsall 1962).

Another alternative, suggested by Friedl (1978), is to employ an Appalachian as ombudsman or liaison to the local community, whose purpose is to increase public awareness of mental health services and provide referrals.

It is also essential to have the input of mountaineers of all class levels in the formulation of mental health service policy and organization. Efforts should be made to achieve broad representation on advisory boards and at public meetings.

5. Familiarize mental health care providers with Appalachian culture. Therapists of non-Appalachian backgrounds need to understand the nature of Appalachian culture in order to effectively provide mental health care. Tolerance of cultural differences is also required. Therapists should also be sensitive to special problems that may afflict mountaineers, such as the stress of modernization and acculturation to mainstream American life.

6. Incorporate a family perspective in mental health care. Given the kin-based nature of Appalachian society, mental health services must begin with the family as the basic unit for health care. It should be recognized, moreover, that the Appalachian family may include extended kin, such as grandparents and married siblings, as significant members outside the household unit. As Herlihy (1963) states, it is essential to get family members' support and endorsement of medical care. If family members are not acknowledged and consulted, they may intervene and prevent successful continuation of treatment.

7. Become involved in mental health research in Appalachia and publish the results. One of the major difficulties in making recommendations for mental health care in Appalachia is the lack of data. There are no published epidemiological studies nor is there much available literature on mental health service utilization rates or response to treatment. Mental health practitioners should begin to document mental health care in the mountains, so that accurate assessments of the services can be made.

REFERENCES

Barrera, M., Jr. 1978. Mexican-American mental health service utilization: A critical examination of some proposed variables. *Community Mental Health Journal* 14 (1):35-45.

Beaver, P.D. 1986. *Rural community in the Appalachian South.* Lexington: University Press of Kentucky.

Burruel, G., and N. Chavez. 1974. Mental health outpatient centers: Relevant or irrelevant to Mexican Americans? In *Beyond clinic walls,* eds. A.B. Tulipan, C.L. Attneave, and E. Kingstone, 108-30. POCA Perspectives No.5. University: University of Alabama Press.

Coles, R. 1967. *Children of Crisis,* vol. 2. *Migrants, sharecroppers, mountaineers.* Boston: Little, Brown.

Friedl, J. 1978. *Health care services and the Appalachian migrant.* Columbus: Ohio State University.

Garrison, V. 1975. Espiritismo: Implications for provision of mental health service to Puerto Rican populations. In *Folk therapy,* eds. H. Hodges and C. Hudson. Miami: University of Miami Press.

Hand, W.D., ed. 1961. *Popular beliefs and superstitions from North Carolina.* The Frank C. Brown Collection of North Carolina Folklore. Durham: Duke University Press.

Herlihy, T.J. 1963. Social work in the southern Appalachians. *American Journal of Public Health* 53:1770-79.

Hicks, G.L. 1976. *Appalachian valley.* New York: Holt, Rinehart & Winston.

Hill, C.E. 1976. A folk medical belief system in the American South: Some practical considerations. *Southern Medicine* 16:11-17.

Hochstrasser, D.L., and G.S. Nickerson. 1966. Community health work in southern Appalachia. *Mountain Life and Work* 42(3):8-16.

Holt, J.B. 1940. Holiness religion: Cultural shock and social reorganization. *American Sociological Review* 5:740-47.

Humphrey, R.A. 1974. Development of religion in southern Appalachia: The personal quality. *Appalachian Journal* 1:244-54.

Kane, S.M. 1974. Ritual possession in a southern Appalachian religious sect. *Journal of American Folklore* 87:293-302.

Kaplan, S.R., and M. Roman. 1973. *The organization and delivery of mental health services in the ghetto: The Lincoln Hospital experience.* New York: Praeger.

Keefe, S.E., A.M. Padilla, and M.L. Carlos. 1979. The Mexican American extended family as an emotional support system. *Human Organization* 38:144-52.

Long, G.M. 1962. Folk medicine in McMinn, Polk, Bradley, and Meigs Counties, Tennessee, 1910-27. *Tennessee Folklore Society Bulletin* 28:1-8.

Looff, D.H. 1971. *Appalachia's children: The challenge of mental health.* Lexington: University Press of Kentucky.

Looff, D.H. 1973. Rural Appalachians and their attitudes toward health. In *Rural and Appalachian Health,* eds. R.L. Nolan & J.L. Schwartz, 3-28. Springfield, Ill.: Charles C Thomas.

Looff, D.H., and M.N. Smith. 1969. School phobia in the southern Appalachian region: Crucial importance of early treatment. *Southern Medical Journal* 62:329-35.

Miller, K.S. 1966. Mental health treatment services and the lower socioeconomic classes. In *Mental health and the lower social classes,* eds. K.S. Miller & C.M. Grigg, 54-61. Tallahassee: Florida State University Press.

Osgood, D., D.L. Hochstrasser, and K.W. Deuschle. 1966. Lay midwifery in southern Appalachia. *Archives of Environmental Health* 12:759-70.

Pearsall, M. 1960. Healthways in a mountain county. *Mountain Life and Work* 35:7-13.

Pearsall, M. 1962. Some behavioral factors in the control of tuberculosis in a rural county. *American Review of Respiratory Diseases* 85:200-10.

Rogers, P.T., and M. Rogers. 1971. A health survey of the pre-school children of Scott County, Tennessee. *Appalachia Medicine* 3:60-64.

Snow, L.F. 1976. "High Blood" is not high blood pressure. *Urban Health* 5:54-55.

Steinman, D. 1970. Health in rural poverty: Some lessons in theory and from experience. *American Journal of Public Health* 60:1813-23.

Stekert, E.J. 1971. Southern mountain medical beliefs in Detroit: Focus for conflict. In *Ethnic Groups in the City*, ed. O. Feinstein, 231-76. Lexington, Mass.: Heath Lexington Books.

Stuart, J. 1966. New wine in old bottles. *Kentucky Folklore Record* 12:105-107.

Tripp-Reimer, T., and M.C. Friedl. 1977. Appalachians: A neglected minority. *Nursing Clinics of North America* 12(1):41-54.

Weller, J.E. 1965. *Yesterday's people: Life in contemporary Appalachia.* Lexington: University of Kentucky Press.

Wigginton, E., ed. 1972. *The foxfire book.* Garden City, N.Y.: Anchor Press/Doubleday.

9

Enhancing the Use of
Mental Health Services

CATHY MELVIN EFIRD

Appalachia's unique social and cultural heritage plays a significant role in the illness behavior of its residents, especially in their decisions to utilize mental health care services. It should play an equally important role in the way mental health care providers plan and deliver mental health services. Too often, mental health personnel fail to consider this unique context and, as a result, find that services are not utilized to the fullest extent possible by the people they are intended to serve.

To enhance the utilization of mental health services in Appalachia, mental health programs themselves must be offered in ways that conform more closely to the special needs of Appalachian people. Understanding the constraints involved in seeking care is necessary to provide a basis for effective changes in mental health care delivery systems. Progress toward these goals can be effectively undertaken through the systematic application of a planning process aimed at eliminating barriers to service utilization. The purpose of this paper is to provide some insight into the planning process itself and into the first step of the process: the task of identifying manipulable factors affecting mental health service utilization in Appalachia.

THE PLANNING PROCESS

The utilization of mental health services in Appalachia has been, and continues to be, hampered by a number of factors considered unique to the region. Historical and cultural forces, especially as they are shaped by fundamentalist religion, dictate the ways in which mental health problems are perceived and the actions taken to alleviate them. Mental health personnel too often fail to consider this context and, as a result, offer what are viewed as inappropriate and unconventional services. Since community mental health centers are not seen as of-

Figure 9.1. The Planning Process.

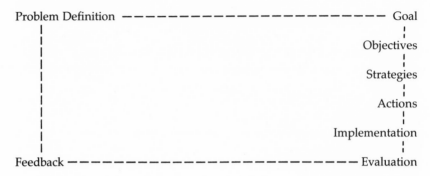

fering viable solutions, they are not considered an acceptable source of care and are not used to the extent that they could be by Appalachian people. If utilization is to be enhanced in Appalachia, if the people truly in need of services are to be reached, then it is essential to explore those factors affecting decisions to seek mental health care. This exploration should be aimed at discovering the particular factors that can be manipulated positively to affect the illness population's behavior and, thereby, mental health service utilization (MacStravic 1978).

Identification of significant barriers to service utilization defines problem areas in service delivery and provides the basis for mental health service planning at the local level. Planning active efforts to correct these problems through policy and resource allocation decisions is a necessary step in providing appropriate and timely mental health services in Appalachia. The planning process itself (see Figure 9.1) begins with the development of a goal or set of goals defined in terms of the problems that have been identified. A goal should state the ultimate aim of the implementation of the planning process. It ought, in other words, to specify the desired long-term outcome of the program. In this case, the overall goal is to improve mental health care utilization in Appalachia. Various subgoals may also be identified as the planning process unfolds.

After this step, practical, achievable objectives that move toward the goals are developed. These objectives should provide a measure of how much progress toward the goal is expected within a certain period of time. Specific time frames and expected levels of achievement are designated for each factor that can be positively manipulated to reduce barriers to service utilization. One objective aimed at enhancing mental health service utilization might be stated as follows:

to increase the number of outpatient mental health services from *(the existing number)* to *(the desired number)* by *(date)*. The quantitative nature of objectives is essential since, without it, objectives remain vague and overall achievement is difficult to assess in the evaluation phase of the planning process. The time frame for objectives is usually longer than that of other plan components, since their achievement generally depends on the successful completion of other tasks.

The question of how to accomplish the objective is addressed in the strategy statements. Like objectives, strategies specify particular tasks that must be undertaken to accomplish the objective and contribute to the long-range goal. Strategies generally have a much shorter time frame and outline program directions for the agency. An example that accompanies this objective might be to develop one satellite clinic in a remote section of the service area by a certain date.

Alternative actions for implementing each strategy are then delineated and evaluated in terms of their cost, the feasibility of implementation, and their expected impact on the overall goal. Those actions that hold the most potential for overcoming barriers to utilization are incorporated into the plan and become a guide for day-to-day agency activities. Implementation of these activities is assigned to particular staff members. As the actions are undertaken and completed, their impact is assessed and used to redefine the utilization problems. In this manner, planning becomes a continuous process aimed at improving mental health service delivery in a constantly changing environment.

The development of a plan in this manner gives each mental health agency a hierarchical guide to the accomplishment of its goals. Each action contributes to the attainment of a strategy, strategies to objectives, and objectives to overall goals. Successful implementation of this type of planning process not only helps the agency achieve its objectives but also provides a practical framework for dealing with new service delivery obstacles as they appear.

A paper such as this cannot begin to substantively outline a mental health plan for Appalachian communities. It can, however, provide some insight into the first step in the planning process: the task of identifying manipulable factors affecting mental health service utilization in Appalachia.

MANIPULABLE FACTORS

Focusing planning efforts on manipulable factors means that some traditional measures of utilization will be of little help in developing the plan. Profiling the client population provides only a certain combination of demographic factors affecting utilization (MacStravic 1978). Although these factors serve a useful function in terms of forecasting utilization trends, they suggest few options for changes that can be affected by policy and resource allocation decisions. Client information also provides a profile of those persons already using mental health services, not of those who still encounter significant barriers to utilization. Decisions to utilize mental health services are affected by two broad categories of manipulable factors. The first of these is the availability of mental health care services, and the second, the accessibility of those services.

The availability of mental health care services has to do primarily with the supply of personnel and facilities. Problems exist when there are too few providers to meet an area's mental health service need or when providers are inappropriately distributed. In Appalachia and other parts of rural America, mental health services as well as primary care services are often unavailable. Three-fourths of the nation's rural counties are designated either in whole or in part as medically underserved areas (Clayton 1978). Although this statistic deals more specifically with primary care, analogous mental health statistics show that 76 percent of counties with less than 100 persons per square mile have no registered psychologist (Keller and Murray 1978). Mental health facilities as well as personnel are also lacking in rural areas of the United States. Only one rural county in fourteen has a general hospital with a psychiatric facility, and only 10 percent of the outpatient psychiatric clinics in the United States are in rural areas (Flax et al. 1979). The proportion of facilities found in rural areas (10 percent) quite clearly does not match the proportion of the population (26 percent) found there (U.S. Bureau of the Census 1983).

Since Appalachia is a predominately rural region, it faces many of the same availability problems. It, too, is underserved in terms of mental health personnel and facilities. According to figures from the Appalachian Regional Commission (ARC), in 1974, only one-half of the 297 Appalachian communities had community mental health centers funded through the National Institute for Mental Health (Swift, Dicker, and McKeown 1975). Furthermore, only 6% of the total ARC expenditure in health went directly to mental health care facilities. Primary care and child development programs funded by the ARC often incorporate a mental health component but the emphasis is clearly on primary health care delivery. Given these statistics, Appalachian communities are very likely to face a shortage of mental health services. This shortage is reflected in both the public and private sectors and thus becomes a concern for the entire community.

Even in the few Appalachian communities where mental health services are readily available, problems often exist in gaining access to those services. Problems with accessibility may be grouped into four general categories: geographical or physical barriers, time barriers, financial barriers, and social barriers. While these barriers may exist within any mental health care system, the specific concerns within each category are often peculiar to a certain locale. Appalachia is no exception to this rule and faces its own barriers to mental health care accessibility. Once again, these barriers form the basis for agency objectives.

Geographically, Appalachia is marked by rugged topography that does not facilitate movement and results in a fairly dispersed settlement pattern. People are more likely to live in the countryside than in towns in most Appalachian counties. This decentralized population, more often than not, is served by a centralized mental health facility. Most community mental health centers are located in the county's largest town or county seat (Steinman 1970). For people living in the countryside, the distance they must travel to reach mental health services is great and presents a substantial barrier to them. Private transportation is the only source available to most Appalachians and its cost as well as inconvenience figure prominently in decisions to seek care. Many researchers have noted the negative effect of distance on primary health care utilization, emphasizing that it often predisposes people to seek curative rather than preventive care and sporadic rather than routine care (Aday and Anderson 1974). The effect of distance in seeking mental health care is probably even more significant since it is often perceived as less essential than other services. Steinman (1970) verifies this conclusion in his study of an Appalachian county's health seeking patterns. He found that geographic isolation and the concentration of services in urban centers were the two most important barriers to service utilization.

The delimitation of catchment areas intensifies geographic barriers in Appalachia. Since designations are based on population and not area, most catchment areas exceed 5000 square miles in size (Clayton 1978). Even a precisely centered facility in an area of that size would be remote for people located on the periphery. Catchment areas also tend to follow political boundaries, such as county lines. In many mountain areas, these boundaries have little meaning since people travel to the nearest facility, whether or not it is in the area defined by catchment designations. Distance once again serves as a barrier to service utilization.

Accessibility may also be defined in terms of the time required to reach a mental health provider and to obtain care. Given the distances that most Appalachian people must travel, the time it takes to get to a facility becomes a significant factor in the decision to utilize services. Under normal circumstances, a U.S. Department of Health, Education and Welfare (HEW) (1977) study found that 20 percent of the rural population had to travel between thirty and sixty minutes to reach their primary source of health care. Travel in Appalachia is anything but normal. Curvy roads that wind around mountains rather than cross them directly add significantly to travel time for rural residents.

In addition to travel time, the amount of time it takes to obtain care must also be considered. Aday and Anderson (1974) cite HEW figures showing that 46 percent of rural nonfarm residents wait at least 30 minutes after arriving in their physician's office. For rural farm residents, this figure rises to 67 percent. This waiting time is almost twice as long as that for the non-central city SMSA residents (75 percent of them saw a physician within thirty minutes of arrival) (Aday and Anderson 1974).

These long travel and waiting times often mean the loss of at least one-half day's work just to keep a mental health appointment. For most wage-earning people and, therefore, most Appalachians, this is time they cannot afford.

Just as time costs can significantly affect decisions to use mental health services, so can the actual cost of obtaining those services. Since health care of all types is still a commodity that must be purchased, poor families enjoy very little in the way of buying power for either the basic commodities of life or for the "luxuries," such as mental health care. Poverty is a way of life for many people in Appalachia. Income levels in the rural areas of the region are 10 to 50 percent lower than the nation (Ford 1962). A band of counties along the North Carolina-Tennessee border has consistently shown lower per capita income figures than the rest of the southern Appalachian region. The family income in these situations, is often less than the national per capita income. Poverty of this magnitude drastically affects a family's or individual's ability to interact with either the public or private mental health care system. This inability to afford care is cited as the third highest factor affecting utilization in the Appalachian county studied by Steinman (1970).

Social service programs provide only limited relief from these economic constraints. Over 40 percent of the poor in rural areas are ineligible for Medicare and Medicaid (Clayton 1978). These people must usually bear the entire cost of obtaining mental health care, since they are employed in low-wage and/or seasonal occupations, which do not provide health insurance as a benefit. Although sliding fee scales help significantly, the addition of an extra expense to the household budget is often seen as a barrier. Appalachia is no exception to this rural pattern and may, in fact, face a more serious situation. The strong family orientation of Appalachian people means families stay together at almost any cost. As intact families, they are often ineligible for health and income support programs, such as Medicaid and Aid to Families with Dependent Children.

Given the high levels of poverty and the inability to qualify for social service programs, Appalachians are confronted with a decision to seek care that centers primarily on economic considerations. The pressure of this expense means that people do not seek care and that when they do, they feel compelled to have a quick solution to their problems. As one informant explained concerning her visits to a local mental health center, "I'm supposed to learn to relax, but when I sit there and realize that I have to pay $15 an hour to relax, I just can't do it." Barriers created by financial concerns threaten not only the utilization of care in this case but also the effectiveness of treatment.

Social barriers to mental health care utilization are also significant manipulable factors. Keefe (Chapter 8) has reviewed the cultural and institutional components of this set of barriers. Cultural factors, or those that can be ascribed to the client, focus on the Appalachian person's definition of mental illness and its causes, as well as the behavior used to modify it. Within this context, Keefe points to the alternative sources of mental health care relied upon by Appalachian residents. Religious, family, and folk medicine interventions are generally pursued prior to contact with the established medical system. Even when the decision has been made to seek professional care, the usual source is the primary care physician rather than the mental health care provider (Lee, Gianturco, and Eisdorfer 1974). The cultural context of Appalachia, then, does not routinely include consideration of mental health services as an alternative source of care for personal problems.

Social factors related to accessibility also include the nature of health service facilities or, what some may term, institutional factors. Keefe (Chapter 8) deals with these barriers in the Appalachian context and identifies two main problem areas. First, social class differences between clients and providers present value conflicts that hamper utilization and render certain techniques ineffective. Young (1977) points to the expectation by Appalachians that mental health care will be like other types of health care: the client describes his or her problem, the expert makes a diagnosis, and the client receives a cure. The client sees no need to "talk" (Young 1977). Verbal therapy in the context of this expectation is clearly inappropriate. Looff (1971) suggests the utility of action-oriented, crisis-model approaches in these situations.

The second set of social barriers centers around communication problems between clients and providers. Regional descriptions of symptoms and reasons offered for them are often not fully understood by mental health care providers. In the same way, suggestions offered by providers may be misunderstood by clients (Keefe, Chapter 8).

These institutional and cultural barriers limit accessibility just as do geographic, time, and financial barriers. To the extent that these barriers are still present in Appalachian communities, accessibility as a problem in mental health service utilization should be dealt with through the planning process. Enhancing accessibility, in these cases, should be a primary subgoal for community mental health centers.

SAMPLE PLAN COMPONENTS

Given these constraints, plans can be developed to address the goal of improved utilization. Objectives that focus on availability and accessibility of mental health services may be written to address each of the constraints and subsequent components added to them.

Increasing the accessibility of mental health services can be translated into a number of objectives. Bodenheimer (1970) suggests that accessible programs should present the client with negligible distance, time, financial, and social barriers to service utilization. The preceding discussion suggests that objectives should focus on reducing these barriers (see Table 9.1). Strategies for meeting the objectives should address the components of those barriers. An agency, for example, may decide to minimize time barriers by staggering appointments so that waiting time is reduced, by locating satellite clinics in outlying areas of the catchment area to reduce driving time, or holding clinics in the evenings or on weekends to reduce time lost from work. Each of the barriers to accessibility can be explored and alternative solutions suggested through the agency's planning process.

This process of identifying manipulable factors affecting mental

Table 9.1. Sample Plan Components.

Goal: To increase the utilization of mental health services in Appalachia.
Subgoal: To increase accessibility of local mental health services in Appalachia.

	Objective 1	Objective 2
Objective	To reduce the average distance clients travel to receive care from ___ to ___ by ___.	To reduce the time involved in seeking and receiving mental health services from ___ to ___ by ___.
Strategy A	To decrease the size of the catchment area from ___ to ___ by ___.	To reduce clinic waiting time from 30 minutes to 15 minutes by ___.
Action 1	Conduct a survey of possible divisions of existing catchment areas.	Establish a standing emergency system to prevent additional waiting.
Action 2	Petition State Mental Health Division for a change in administrative structure of catchment area.	Increase the number of staff members dealing directly with clients.
Strategy B	Decentralize mental health facilities by locating at least one facility in a remote area of the county by ___.	To reduce driving time from ___ to ___ by ___.
Action 1	Initiate a site selection process.	Offer outpatient services on site at major industrial sites.
Action 2	Seek necessary funds through grantswriting, fundraising, etc.	
Strategy C	To reduce time lost from work from ___ to ___.	
Action 1	Establish evening and weekend hours.	
Action 2	Consolidate family member visits, if possible.	

health service utilization and of developing plans to deal with them can provide local communities and local mental health centers with a systematic approach to solving their problems. It must be remembered that this is a cooperative process and that plans must be developed by each agency in conjunction with the community members affected by those problems. Members of advisory boards and councils do not, typically, fulfill this role. It is often necessary to provide a different structure for community input into the planning process. Small task forces composed of agency personnel, clients, and potential clients could be organized around each problem area and given the responsibility of developing certain plan components. This structure provides an opportunity to include all types of community members as a supplement to the existing board. Each community then has the ability to develop a plan that addresses the unique utilization barriers facing it and the flexibility to deal with new issues in a timely manner.

REFERENCES

Aday, L.A., and R. Anderson. 1974. *Development of indices of access to medical care.* Ann Arbor: Health Administration Press, University of Michigan.

Bodenheimer, T.S. 1970. Patterns of American ambulatory care. *Inquiry* 7(3):26-37.

Clayton, T. 1978. Issues in the delivery of rural mental health services. *Hospital and Community Psychiatry* 28(9): 673-76.

Flax, J.W., O. Morton, R.E. Wagenfeld, R.E. Ivens, and R.J. Weiss. 1979. *Mental health and rural America: An overview and annotated bibliography.* Washington, D.C.: U.S. Government Printing Office.

Ford, T.R., ed. 1962. *The southern Appalachian region: A survey.* Lexington: University of Kentucky Press.

Keller, P.A., and J.D. Murray. 1978. Psychology and rural America: An overview. Mansfield, Pa.: Department of Psychology.

Lee, S.H., D.T. Gianturco, and C. Eisdorfer. 1974. Community mental health center accessibility: A survey of the rural poor. *Archives of General Psychiatry* 31:335-39.

Looff, D.H. 1971. *Appalachia's children: The challenge of mental health.* Lexington: University Press of Kentucky.

MacStravic, R.E. 1978. *Determining health needs.* Ann Arbor: Health Administration Press, University of Michigan.

Steinman, D. 1970. Health in rural poverty: Some lessons in theory and from experience. *American Journal of Public Health* 60:1813-23.

Swift, B., R. Dicker, and M. McKeown. 1975. Mental health in Appalachia: An emerging problem. *Appalachia* (October-November):36-44.

U.S. Bureau of the Census. 1983. *Characteristics of the population: General social and economic characteristics: U.S. summary, 1980,* Table 182, pp. 1-180. Washington, D.C.: U.S. Government Printing Office.

U.S. Department of Health, Education and Welfare. 1977. *Health of the disadvantaged: Chartbook.* DHEW Pub. No. (HRA) 77-628. Washington, D.C.: U.S. Government Printing Office.

Young, B. 1977. Appalachian women and mental health: A discussion. *Mountain Life and Work* (November-December):13-15.

10

An Exploratory Study of Mental Health Service Utilization by Appalachians and Non-Appalachians

SUSAN EMLEY KEEFE

Mental health services in Appalachia must serve more and more diverse populations. No longer is the region a hinterland where traditional life endures relatively unchanged, made up of more or less homogeneous face-to-face communities. Nor has Appalachia remained a region of economic decline and out-migration. On the contrary, southern Appalachia's population grew by 19 percent between 1970-1980 (Pickard 1981). Growth was particularly significant in those parts of southern Appalachia with economies based primarily on tourism and recreation, vacation homes, and retirement populations. Those moving into the region include return migrants and newcomers from all parts of the United States, even from outside the country.

The newcomers in Appalachia are different in origins. Some come from the South, some from the North. National heritage and religious affiliation are heterogeneous. On the other hand, some commonalities emerge: most are white, middle class, and have an urban background. Newcomers, furthermore, tend to be mainstream Americans, following the cultural norms typically cited as American.

Newcomers are changing the Appalachian scene. They have a different attitude toward the land and the use of land (Stephenson 1984). Differences in values between newcomers and Appalachian natives can cause social conflict and political realignment (Keefe 1983). In some ways, newcomers and natives can be seen as distinctive groups that compete for resources in the public arena. One important resource is encompassed by health and mental health services. Comparison of aspects of mental health service utilization by ethnic groups is common in the mental health literature (e.g., Andrulis 1977; Sue 1977; Tischler et al. 1975). This paper presents an exploratory study of mental health service utilization data comparing native Appalachians with non-Appalachian newcomers. The findings demonstrate differences in utilization rates, the clients' sociocultural and economic background, and clinic referral and treatment. The results confirm the need to think in cultural terms when developing and implementing services for the Appalachian region.

METHOD OF ANALYSIS

Data were obtained for the New River Mental Health District which covers five mountain counties in western North Carolina: Alleghany, Ashe, Avery, Watauga, and Wilkes. The state of North Carolina, Division of Mental Health Services, supplies a uniform "fact sheet" or data collection form to all public mental health clinics in the state. The form provides for the collection of data regarding each client, including admission, program tracking, and termination data. These data are analyzed statistically each year by the state and results are provided to the local districts.

Information on birthplace is used in this study for the purpose of identification of clients as Appalachian natives versus non-Appalachians. Data on birthplace was collected by the state from 1975 through July 1979, at which time it became an optional item and many mental health service agencies including New River opted to drop the question. Therefore, the data analyzed herein are limited to clients utilizing local mental health services during the period 1975-1979. The sample is further limited by the manner in which birthplace data were collected. While the county of birth was requested of North Carolina-born clients, no specification of county was required if birth was outside the state. Thus, it is impossible to determine Appalachian birth in the remaining eleven states where only a portion is considered Appalachian.[1] For the purpose of this study, therefore, Appalachian natives are defined as those clients born in the Appalachian counties of North Carolina or in the state of West Virginia and non-Appalachians are defined as those clients born in the non-Appalachian counties of North Carolina and in non-Appalachian states. Fourteen percent of the sample of terminated clients was eliminated by the way in which birthplace was ultimately defined. Over one-third of the eliminated portion of the original sample of clients were born in the adjacent states of Virginia and Tennessee and most likely are Appalachian natives. The final sample from the five-county district totals 5140; the alcohol detox center sample for the five counties totals

Table 10.1. 1975-1979 Mental Health Service Utilization Rate (by birthplace of client)

Facility Utilized	Appalachian		Non-Appalachian		Undetermined	
	N	%	N	%	N	%
Alcohol detox	1110	90	47	4	80	6
Alleghany	227	68	56	14	74	18
Ashe	484	75	54	8	108	17
Avery	582	71	127	15	114	14
Watauga	933	57	356	22	334	21
Wilkes	1985	80	286	12	206	8
5-County Total	4261	71	879	15	836	14

Source: New River Mental Health Services data on terminated clients.

1157. These two samples are analyzed separately given the different nature of the treatment population and services received.

Table 10.1 presents mental health service utilization data for the five counties and the single alcohol detox center serving these counties by client's birthplace. Data for the portion of the sample for which Appalachian birthplace could not be determined are included to provide a more complete picture of utilization. An average of 15 percent of the clients served by the five county facilities are non-Appalachians; Ashe County serves the lowest proportion of non-Appalachians (8 percent) whereas Watauga County serves the highest proportion (22 percent). Significantly, only a very small proportion (4 percent) of clients using the alcohol detox facility are non-Appalachians.

Comparative statistics on birthplace in the general population are not available. The U.S. Bureau of the Census does not break down population statistics by birthplace except for the foreign-born population. Regional planners (using migration data), however, estimate that almost 70 percent of the population growth in the North Carolina mountains from 1970-1980 was made up of newcomers (Hammersly and Henderson 1983). In Watauga County, a tourist center and the location of a large state university, for example, the population grew by 35 percent between 1970-1980 and 82 percent of this was the result of migration. In other words, 21 percent of the county's population in 1980 were recent migrants. How many of these recent migrants are returning Appalachian natives or immigrants from other Appalachian

Table 10.2. Comparison of Appalachian and Non-Appalachian Status of Mental Health Clinic Clients and the General Population

	1975-1979 Mental Health Service Clients[a]		1980 General Population		
County	Appalachian (N = 4261) %	Non-Appalachian (N = 879) %	Base 1970 Population %	Natural Increase %	In-Migration %
Alleghany	83	17	85	2	13
Ashe	90	10	87	4	9
Avery	82	18	88	5	7
Watauga	72	28	74	5	21
Wilkes	87	13	84	7	9
5-County Total	83	17	83	5	12

Sources: New River Mental Health Services and Region D Council of Governments.
[a]These figures are based on the total number of terminated clients whose birthplace could be determined.

areas versus non-Appalachian born migrants is impossible to determine without further information, however. It is not known, moreover, what proportion of the 1970 population was native versus non-Appalachian. Considering the recent turnaround in Appalachian migration from greater out-migration to greater in-migration, it could be assumed that the proportion of non-Appalachians present in 1970 was fairly small.

Recognizing these problems, but for purposes of gross comparison, Table 10.2 presents a breakdown of mental health service clients and the general population by birthplace or migration status. Since the data on the general population is from 1980, the percentage of in-migrants in the general population is probably higher than it would have been over the period of 1975-1979 covered by the mental health services data. This is probably balanced, on the other hand, by the fact that some proportion of the 1970 population was made up of in-migrants. Taking the percentages at face value, it is apparent that non-Appalachians are more likely than Appalachian natives to use mental health services. The greater likelihood runs from a low of 1 percent in Ashe County, where recent in-migrants make up 9 percent of the population and 10 percent of the mental health clients are non-

Appalachians, to a high of 11 percent in Avery County, where in-migrants make up 7 percent of the population and 18 percent of the mental health clients are non-Appalachians. According to the five county average, only 12 percent of the population are in-migrants but 17 percent of the mental health clinic users are non-Appalachians.

The corollary finding is that Appalachian natives underutilize mental health services. Underutilization by subgroups is sometimes explained by proposing these subgroups have fewer emotional problems, but more likely it indicates some irrelevance of mental health services for the subgroups and an inability to compete equally for the services (Keefe, Chapter 8; Keefe and Casas 1980). These findings indicate the need for greater attention to mental health service utilization in Appalachia and the impact on utilization of increased migration into the region. It may be that as the proportion of newcomers increases, as seems likely, Appalachian natives may be less and less likely to be able to compete for and receive adequate mental health care.

COMPARISON OF APPALACHIAN AND
NON-APPALACHIAN CLIENTS

Clients of Appalachian and non-Appalachian descent using the five mental health centers and the alcohol detox center were compared on the following characteristics: age, sex, race, marital status, number in the household, living arrangement, and education. Statistical significance was evaluated using chi-square; if the probability was 5 percent or less, it was accepted as significant. Differences emerged between Appalachian and non-Appalachian clients and between mental health center clients and alcohol detox center clients.

Mental health clinic users are fairly homogeneous by race. The vast majority of both Appalachian and non-Appalachian clients are white (97 percent) much like the local population at large. Most of the non-whites are blacks; there are few American Indian, Asian, or Hispanic residents in the area.

Both non-Appalachian and Appalachian mental health clients are likely to be women, but there is a significant difference in the proportion of the sexes in the two groups. Non-Appalachian clients are much more likely to be women (60 percent women vs. 40 percent men) while Appalachian clients are only somewhat more likely to be women (53 percent women vs. 47 percent men).

There is also a significant difference by age. Although the majority of clients in both groups are under thirty-six years of age, Appalachian clients are more likely to be middle aged, that is, 36 to 59 years of age, than non-Appalachians (33 percent vs. 21 percent). Reasons for the significant age and sex differences between Appalachian and non-Appalachian clients are not immediately apparent, and further research is needed to explain why men and the middle aged, who suffer least in the general population, seem to be more at risk in Appalachia.

The majority of clients in both groups are not married. Statistical tests of significance, however, demonstrate that Appalachians are somewhat more likely to be married (42 percent vs. 39 percent) while non-Appalachians are somewhat more likely to be single (44 percent vs. 39 percent).

The more familistic nature of Appalachians is also evident in the data on living arrangements. Appalachians are more likely to be living with relatives (spouse, children, and other kin) than non-Appalachians (84 percent vs. 70 percent). Although only 20 percent of the Appalachian clients are less than eighteen years of age, 34 percent of them live with their parents; in comparison, 20 percent of the non-Appalachian clients are also less than eighteen years old, but only 26 percent live with their parents. There is no significant difference between the two groups in number living in the household.

Additional data indicate that Appalachians are less geographically mobile, which further contributes to their familism. Only 4 percent of the Appalachian clients were terminated due to having moved compared to 13 percent of the non-Appalachians. Geographic stability is also indicated by the birthplace data: an average of 55 percent of the Appalachian clients were born in the county in which they used a mental health clinic.

According to the education data, Appalachian natives have significantly lower levels of education than non-Appalachians. While 20 percent of both groups are under eighteen years of age, fully one-third of the Appalachians have only eight years of education or less compared to only 16 percent of the non-Appalachians. Fifty-eight percent of the Appalachians have not graduated from high school compared to 33 percent of the non-Appalachians. Barely 8 percent of the Appalachians have been to college compared to 31 percent of the non-Appalachians. Appalachian clients clearly are not only a distinct cultural group, they also differ socioeconomically from non-Appalachians; the majority of Appalachian clients are working class or lower class. Moreover, Appalachians are somewhat more likely to be unemployed (26 percent vs. 21 percent).

Clients at the alcohol detox facility are racially similar to the mental health clinic users, the vast majority being white. Detox clients, however, differ by age and sex. While mental health clinic users tend to be women, alcohol detox clients are overwhelmingly men (98 percent). Detox clients also tend to be somewhat older than the clinic users; the majority of detox clients are thirty-six years of age or older while the majority of clinic users are less than thirty-six years old.

There are age and sex differences between Appalachian and non-Appalachian detox clients that, while not reaching statistical significance, are of interest. Appalachian women are least likely to be admitted to the detox facility; only 2 percent of the Appalachian detox clients are women compared to 6 percent of the non-Appalachians. Appalachian detox clients tend to be younger than the non-Appalachian clients; 27 percent of the Appalachians are under 36 years of age as opposed to only 13 percent of the non-Appalachians.

Detox clients and mental health clinic users differ by marital status. While mental health users are equally likely to be married or single, detox clients are most likely to be married or separated or divorced. There are no statistically significant differences between Appalachian and non-Appalachian detox clients on marital status, but it is interesting to note that non-Appalachians are somewhat more likely than Appalachians to be married (53 percent vs. 44 percent) and Appalachians are more likely than non-Appalachians to be separated (14 percent vs. 6 percent).

According to data on living arrangements, detox clients are more likely than mental health clinic users to live alone (27 percent vs. 7 percent). There is no significant difference between Appalachian and non-Appalachian detox clients in living arrangements. A comparison of Appalachian clients at the detox facility versus the mental health clinic indicates less familistic living arrangements among the detox clients; in particular, fewer detox clients live with relatives other than spouse and children. There is no significant difference between Appalachians and non-Appalachians in number living in the household, but in general, detox clients live in somewhat smaller households than the mental health clinic users.

Finally, with regard to education, alcohol detox clients have lower levels of education than mental health clinic users in general, and a majority of both Appalachians (68 percent) and non-Appalachians (62 percent) have not graduated from high school. It continues to be the case, however, that Appalachian clients have significantly lower levels of education than non-Appalachians. For example, 42 percent of the

Appalachian detox clients have only had eight years of education or less compared to 21 percent of the non-Appalachian clients; 21 percent of the non-Appalachians have had some college compared to only 7 percent of the Appalachians. Appalachian clients, furthermore, are more likely than non-Appalachians to be unemployed (34 percent vs. 26 percent).

In summary, both Appalachian and non-Appalachian mental health clinic users tend to be similar in race and marital status but they differ in other ways. Non-Appalachian clients tend to be young women and fairly well-educated. Appalachian clients, on the other hand, come from a broader spectrum of the population and are more likely to include men as well as women, the middle-aged as well as the young. Appalachian clients in general have fairly low levels of education and are more family oriented. Among detox clients, Appalachians and non-Appalachians are more similar, being typically white working- or lower-class middle-aged men, married now or sometime in the past. Appalachian detox clients are somewhat more likely to be young men, and they have even lower levels of education than the non-Appalachians. Appalachian detox clients, in addition, differ significantly from Appalachian mental health clinic users by being more isolated and less familistic. These intergroup and intragroup differences indicate that cultural background is an important variable in patterns of mental health service utilization in southern Appalachia. More research is required to better interpret the nature of these cultural differences and their impact on the use of mental health services.

Analysis of the data on referral and treatment indicate Appalachians and non-Appalachians pursue different pathways to mental health centers and are treated differently once they arrive.

According to the data on referral agents for mental health clinic users, individuals and health facilities are the two most common referral agents for both Appalachians and non-Appalachians (see Table 10.3). Appalachians, however, are less likely than non-Appalachians to indicate an individual (45 percent vs. 56 percent), whereas Appalachians are more likely than non-Appalachians to indicate a health facility (23 percent vs. 17 percent). In fact, although individuals are most likely to be referral agents for non-Appalachians, agencies or services in general tend to refer Appalachians. Self-referral rates, for example, are higher for non-Appalachins than for Appalachians (29 percent vs. 22 percent). Interestingly, there is little difference between the two subgroups in referral by relatives or friends. Appalachians,

Table 10.3. Comparison of Referral Agents for Appalachians and Non-Appalachians to Mental Health and Detox Centers

Referral Agent	Mental Health Clinics		Alcohol Detox Center	
	Appalachian (N = 4261) %	Non-Appalachian (N = 879) %	Appalachian (N = 1086) %	Non-Appalachian (N = 47) %
Individuals	45	56	69	72
Self	22	29	32	36
Relatives	10	11	1	0
Friends	3	7	1	0
Other	10	9	35	36
Health Facilities	23	17	13	13
Physician	20	14	3	2
General hospital	1	1	3	2
Other	2	3	7	9
Psychiatric and Mental Health Facilities	10	4	9	9
Community mental health center	1	1	8	9
Public mental hospital	5	2	0	0
Other	5	2	1	0
Forensic	12	9	7	2
Justice	5	5	5	2
Court	6	4	1	0
Police	1	0	2	0
Other	1	1	1	0
Human Resources Agencies	5	3	1	0
Social service agency	4	3	1	0
Other	1	1	0	0
Other Residential Facilities	2	6	0	0
Geriatric boarding care	2	6	0	0
Other	1	0	0	0
Other Services or Agencies	3	4	<1	4
Education	3	3	0	0
Clergy	1	1	1	2
Alcoholics Anonymous	1	1	1	2
Other	1	0	0	0

Source: New River Mental Health Services data on terminated clients, 1975-1979.
Note: Totals may include multiple referrals of individual client.

on the other hand, are more likely than non-Appalachians to be referred by a physician. In sum, the data indicate that Appalachians are less likely to come to mental health services through informal pathways, which could mean that mental health services are perceived less positively by Appalachians. The fact that one-fifth of the Appalachians are at the mental health clinic on the advice of a physician indicates the importance of doctors in the helping networks of Appalachians and the need to more fully integrate physicians into the mental health system to better reach Appalachian people. Despite the importance of religion in the culture, on the other hand, it is instructive to note the unlikelihood of religious leaders to refer clients (less than 1 percent) to mental health services. This is quite likely due to a number of cultural values: the tendency to see preachers as equals rather than as authority figures; the reticence of clergy to give unwanted advice; the likelihood of keeping personal problems within the family.

Data on referral agents for clients using the alcohol detox center do not show striking differences between Appalachians and non-Appalachians (see Table 10.3). Most of these clients have individual referral agents, but Appalachians have a somewhat greater chance of arriving at the detox center through the forensic system, that is, the justice system and the police.

Diagnosis is a difficult category to evaluate given problems in definition of categories and differences in application from therapist to therapist. Nevertheless, cumulative differences do appear in comparing the diagnoses of Appalachians and non-Appalachians (see Table 10.4). There is no difference in the diagnosis of mental retardation, organic brain syndrome, psychosis, or psychophysiological illness. Appalachians, however, are more likely to have diagnoses of neurosis and personality disorder (33.7 percent vs. 25.5 percent) while non-Appalachians are more likely to have the less severe diagnoses of transient situational disturbance and behavior disorder (42.6 percent vs. 27.5 percent). This finding parallels other research on mental health clinic utilization by ethnic minorities, who are diagnosed differently and more severely ill than white mainstream clients (Sue 1977). It would be useful to know the birthplace and subgroup status of the diagnosticians at the five mental health centers studied in order to evaluate the effect of any client-therapist cultural difference on diagnosis as well as treatment. This information, unfortunately, is not available. It has been suggested that health and mental health professionals in Appalachia are quite likely to be nonnatives (see Plaut,

Table 10.4. Comparison of Diagnosis at Intake of Mental Health Clinic
Clients

Diagnosis	Appalachian (N = 4261) %	Non-Appalachian (N = 879) %
Mental retardation	1.4	1.2
Organic brain syndrome	2.4	2.2
Psychosis	8.5	8.8
Neurosis	16.6	11.0
Personality disorder	17.1	14.5
Psychophysiological	1.0	0.8
Transient situational	18.0	29.1
Behavior disorder	9.5	13.5
Other	25.5	17.6

Source: New River Mental Health Services data on terminated clients, 1975-1979.

Chapter 11).[2] The mental health literature on ethnic minorities abundantly indicates that, where cultural disparity exists between client and therapist, differences in perception of normal-abnormal arise, ultimately affecting the diagnostic procedure (Karno and Edgerton 1969; Torrey 1972). Rather than indicating that Appalachians are more likely to be more severely mentally ill, the results here could simply reflect cultural miscommunication in the diagnostic process.

Another indication of cultural difference in illness rate is the breakdown of clients by subgroup at the alcohol detox center, where 96 percent are Appalachian natives, while only 83 percent of the mental health clinic users and 88 percent of the general population are natives. It is unclear exactly why Appalachians are more likely to use the detox center. Alcoholism rates could be higher for Appalachians than non-Appalachians. According to the diagnostic data on the mental health clinic users, Appalachians are somewhat more likely to be diagnosed alcoholic (11 percent vs. 6 percent). Perhaps due primarily to their lower social status, Appalachians are also apparently more likely to get caught up in the institutional system that deals with misconduct associated with alcoholism (e.g., the police, justice system) and, thus, they are more likely to be so labeled.

There is some indication that Appalachians are less likely to receive full treatment in a mental health clinic; for example, they are more likely than non-Appalachians to terminate treatment after the initial contact (29 percent vs. 24 percent). This could be due to cultural differences in expectations about the services or differences in the type of services received or differences in need.

To summarize, Appalachian mental health clients are referred to the clinic through formal agencies or services, are likely to receive a more severe diagnosis at the clinic, and are somewhat less likely to continue treatment after the initial contact. Non-Appalachians, on the other hand, come to the clinic through informal referrals and are likely to receive a less severe diagnosis. Aside from the influence of cultural perception of normal-abnormal on the diagnostic process, the more severe diagnosis for Appalachians could also be the result of the formal pathway to help, in which only more severe and persistent symptoms bring about referrals. Appalachian detox clients are somewhat more likely to be referred by the legal system, also indicating more formal pathways to treatment. The greater likelihood that Appalachians become detox clients could thus be related to their relationship to institutional systems in general, as well as indicating a potentially higher incidence of alcoholism.

The data presented in this paper indicate important differences between Appalachian natives and non-Appalachians in mental health service utilization. The results are very similar to utilization studies comparing ethnic minorities with mainstream Americans. Appalachian natives appear to underutilize public mental health clinics. As mental health clients, Appalachians are more familistic and come from a lower socioeconomic background. They reach mental health services through institutional rather than informal networks, and they are likely to be diagnosed as more severely mentally ill. Furthermore, data on the use of the alcohol detox center indicate a higher rate of utilization by Appalachians. The reasons for these differences between Appalachians and non-Appalachians are by no means readily apparent. I have suggested various explanations that could account for these differences, but clearly, more empirical research is needed.

The fact that Appalachian clients tend to differ in cultural and socioeconomic background from non-Appalachians indicates the need to consider alternative forms of therapy when serving both groups. Some therapeutic models and approaches may work well with one group but not the other, or certain forms of therapy may be particularly suited to one group or the other. It would seem, for example, that family therapy would work especially well with Appalachians considering their intensive family orientation (see Cole, Chapter 12).

In areas of southern Appalachia where in-migration is high, mental health clinics will need to make a special effort to ensure that all subpopulations receive adequate services. Not to recognize the distinctiveness of subgroups served will only lead to inequitable service delivery.

One way in which to monitor mental health service utilization by Appalachians and non-Appalachians is to record birthplace information (by county and state) for all clients. This should be a part of the admissions data taken by every mental health facility in the Appalachian region. Similarly, birthplace information from therapists would also be important. Data of this kind would permit more extensive analysis of intergroup and intragroup differences and would permit important long-term studies of utilization in regions of rapid demographic change. Mental health professionals in the Appalachian region should be encouraged to support this kind of research at their own agencies.

NOTES

The author gratefully acknowledges the help of Dr. David Johnson, research psychologist with New River Mental Health, without whom this study could not have been completed. Johnson made the data accessible and helped in the interpretation of the data collection instrument and the intergroup analysis. Data manipulation was performed by the N.C. Division of Mental Health Services.

1. Appalachian counties are defined in this study using the ARC boundaries of the region (The new Appalachian subregions 1974). Only the state of West Virginia lies wholly within the Appalachian region, which also includes parts of Alabama, Georgia, Kentucky, Maryland, Mississippi, New York, Ohio, Pennsylvania, South Carolina, Tennessee, and Virginia.

2. At the workshop on Appalachian mental health that gave impetus to this volume, only 23 percent of the mental health professionals attending were Appalachian natives.

REFERENCES

Andrulis, D.P. 1977. Ethnicity as a variable in the utilization and referral patterns of a comprehensive mental health center. *Journal of Community Psychology* 5:231-37.

Hammersly, L., and B. Henderson. 1983. Two cultures struggle for control of N.C. mountains. *Charlotte Observer* (March 27):1.

Karno, M., and R.B. Edgerton. 1969. Perception of mental illness in a Mexican-American community. *Archives of General Psychiatry* 20(2):233-38.

Keefe, S.E. 1983. Ethnic conflict in an Appalachian craft cooperative: On the application of structural ethnicity to mountaineers and outsiders. In *The Appalachian Experience*, eds. B.M. Buxton, M.L. Crutchfield, W.E. Lightfoot, and J.P. Stewart, 15-25. Boone, N.C.: Appalachian Consortium Press.

Keefe, S.E., and J.M. Casas. 1980. Mexican Americans and mental health: A selected review and recommendations for mental health service delivery. *American Journal of Community Psychology* 8:303-26.

The new Appalachian subregions and their development strategies. 1974. *Appalachia* 8(1):11-27.

Pickard, J. 1981. Appalachia's decade of change = A decade of immigration. *Appalachia* 15(1):24-28.

Stephenson, J. 1984. Escape to the periphery: Commodifying place in rural Appalachia. *Appalachian Journal* 11:187-200.

Sue, S. 1977. Community mental health services to minority groups: Some optimism, some pessimism. *American Psychologist* 32: 616-24.

Tischler, G.L., J.E. Henisz, J.K. Myers, and P.C. Boswell. 1975. Utilization of mental health services: II. Mediators of service allocation. *Archives of General Psychiatry* 32:416-18.

Torrey, E.F. 1972. *The mind game: Witchdoctors and psychiatrists.* New York: Emerson Hall Publishers.

PART IV

Cultural Considerations in Therapeutic Encounters

11

Cross-Cultural Conflict between Providers and Clients and Staff Members

THOMAS PLAUT

In mental health work we are often reminded that one ought to "start where the client is." Experience suggests, however, that this is not so easy to do; that, as sensitive as we might try to be, culture runs deeper than the awareness we carry in everyday life. The ways we move, talk, listen, dress, stand and sit, and make decisions are all symbols to be interpreted by others around us. In the social world of the urban professional, there seems to be a broad consensus as to the meaning of gesture and symbols that form a part of our world taken for granted. The thesis presented here is that this consensus is not generally shared by many of the rural folk who live on the fringes of urban mass culture and retain distinctive world views and symbolic interpretations, often not understood by the practitioner. The lack of common understanding among the urban professionals and local staff members and clients can, and in my experience has, seriously weakened health service delivery programs in Appalachia.

Ethnocentrism and the inability to perceive the significance and validity of variant symbols and modes of being is apparent in the literature on community health systems. Houpt, Orleans, George and Brodie's (1979) study on *The Importance of Mental Health Services to General Health Care*, for example, examines the variables of age, sex, and illness but does not consider the cultural milieu in which these exist. Common texts such as the *Manual for the Comprehensive Community Mental Health Clinic* (Knight and Davis 1969) suffer from the same myopia (see also Glasscote, Sanders, Forstenzer, and Foley 1964; Mechanic, 1979). The call for cultural sensitivity seems to come from those involved with providing or studying the provision of care to a specific minority, such as blacks or Mexican Americans (Duran 1975; Keefe and Casas 1980; Thomas and Comer 1973; Torrey 1970).

The data in this paper come from interviews with the staff members of a mental health center and a primary medical care program in a predominantly rural Appalachian county in western North Carolina. The county is poor: per capita income in 1980 was just 57% of the national average. Industrial wages are low; it ranked in the high seventies among North Carolina's 100 counties in terms of average weekly earning of insured workers (Carlisle and Monteith 1983). In early 1980, I conducted a series of interviews with the staff members of the primary care health program at the request of the director, who said "the consensus seems to be that we need someone to come in and work with us. The issues are not really all that clear in the minds of the staff, other than to desire an improvement in the work setting, particularly around communication!" The staff was divided into three groups: nonprofessionals (clerks, receptionists, van drivers, etc.), which included 17 people; midlevel professionals (nurses, family nurse practitioners, physicians assistants, and a social worker), numbering seven people; and, finally, the professionals (two doctors and a dentist). Several discussions were also held with the program director. Virtually all the professionals and midlevel professionals came from outside the county and the Appalachian region, whereas the nonprofessionals were native to the area. (This, of course, mirrors an all-too-familiar form of stratification in Appalachia as well as other "peripheral" areas.) All participants were administered the Twenty Statements Test and a questionnaire designed to reveal significant others. Neither vehicle found dramatic differences between groups, although some clues assisted the group interview process. About seven hours were spent in discussion with the local nonprofessionals, about three with the midlevel professionals, and two with the professionals. The consultation ended with a morning-long encounter session including the entire staff, which focused on the pervasive difficulties that had surfaced between local and nonlocal, or inmigrant staff members.

The findings of this exercise in research and problem solving have been echoed by other students of the Appalachian region (Lewis 1971; Friedl 1979). In presenting the data at a May 1983 Workshop on Rural Mental Health in North Carolina: Social Work Practice and Ethnocultural Issues, I found sufficient commonality between the world views of rural mountain people and rural blacks to suspect that much of the findings may have an even broader applicability to rural people, rather than just a particular situation or region. On the other hand, the dangers of this sort of generalization require caution, as variance is always found among groups and communities.

My focus here will center on differences in patterns of interaction and in interpretation of behavior and symbols between the practitioners who are products of the urban American mainstream and the support staff members who are rural people of the southern mountains. My research indicates six general areas that are problematic in relations: (1) labeling (how people define and refer to each other), (2) orientation in interaction, (3) definitions of *time*, (4) approaches to problem solving, (5) interpretations of change, and (6) God and the role of the sacred in everyday life.

One prefatory note: the media, through comics such as "Snuffy Smith" or television programs like "The Dukes of Hazard," have given rural Americans and especially those in the southern mountains the idea that their urban compatriots see them in shallow and stereotypic terms. A colleague suggests labels such as *briar* and *hick* have led to an Appalachian love-hate relationship with urban things and people. This relationship makes mountain people wary in any encounter with persons defined as not from around here. A practitioner in a mental or physical health setting is most effective when that wariness is overcome. This happens as the practitioner establishes herself or himself as a person who can comfortably function in and respect the clients' world. Several practices by practitioners inhibit establishing rapport with clients.

LABELING: HOW DO PEOPLE REFER TO EACH OTHER?

A receptionist called to a client sitting in the waiting room of a mental health center. "Mr. Johnson, would you . . ." "When you call me that I just don't feel like it's me," the client responded.

In this example, the formality and impersonalism implied by the use of the last name seemed incongruous to the client, who was accustomed to the individual, personal identity that accompanies the use of first names in his rural mountain community. A similar problem arose at the Southern Mountain Health Program (a pseudonym), when federal government consultants called the use of first names in interactions between staff and clients unprofessional. One local staff member said in an interview: "I can't call someone I've grown up with *mister*. I see him all the time. We go to church together. If I call him mister, when I got off work he'd say to me, 'what's wrong with you? You gettin' a big head up there at the clinic?' I just can't do it."

Practitioners coming to rural areas soon learn that in small communities individuals see themselves and others as having individual, particular identities as opposed to seeing themselves as rooted in a group or category of people. These identities are given or ascribed, not achieved. A rural client told me: "Our preacher was going to go to school to study the Bible. But people in our community got real concerned that he might try to become a preacher, instead of being one . . . that learning about the word of God would stop him from hearing it, and he might not be called to God anymore."

Anthropologist Helen Lewis writes of asking the rural lad "Johnny" what he plans to be when he grows up. His answer is "Johnny" (Lewis 1971, p. 6). He sees himself as a recognized individual within the group with rights, duties, and obligations. What he may ultimately do for a living is secondary.

ORIENTATIONS IN INTERACTION

As an extension of the point just made, in impersonal, urban social systems, structural anonymity requires us to tell people who we are. We continually present ourselves: our legitimacy and status in the social system requires it. (Take a moment sometime to watch how students greet a maintenance man on campus as opposed to a teacher. Do they give any recognition to the existence of the former?) We learn very early in life that we must expend considerable energy presenting ourselves in the urban world. Our legitimacy, we are taught, depends on our achieved status. We make certain that people know we are social workers, therapists, teachers, graduate students, or whatever. In rural social systems, however, status is not achieved by the individual but ascribed by the community. Persons who seek recognition on the basis of achievement or position are often criticized for "gettin' above their raisin' " (Matthews 1966, p. 75). The one notable exception is the medical doctor, whose position in the community clearly is based on achieved status.

From Georg Simmel to Erving Goffman, microsociologists have observed how people present themselves to obtain legitimacy and control in social situations. Such presentations invariably require some skill in verbal communication. The communication itself is often seen as a kind of "chatter" offensive in the rural cultural world; people who talk about themselves are seen as trying to stand out from rather than fit into the group (Hicks 1976). Additionally, the chatter is also symbolic of a skill and agility with words that many rural people find threatening. "They can out-talk you, and out-think you," one local informant said. A clinic receptionist told me, "The director is always talking in words that go over my head. Big, long words. With him you have to be very clever . . . you have to play at putting words together in various ways." Implied in statements such as this is the idea that insufficient cleverness leads to vulnerability and being manipulated. Anxiety and resentment was notably associated with the receptionist's dictum "you have to play." One informant complained: "Why, they don't even know how to be quiet! If it's quiet before a meeting, Mr. G [an administrator] can't stand it. He gets real nervous." Another emphasized the value placed on nonverbal behavior and interaction. "You don't need to talk all the time. Why you can plant a field and never say a word."

There's another danger in those chattering urban professionals in the eyes of a rural client: they don't know how to listen. "They don't know how to listen to us. We know this area. *We're from here*. We know how people feel and what's going on." A receptionist commented on doctors: "They don't listen to the patients . . . *they just ask questions but don't really listen* . . . they make us feel like we just don't understand, or that whatever it is is our fault."

The perception of not listening leads to an interpretation of assumed superiority on the part of the other party and, additionally, to the idea that the professional doesn't really care about the client. If these perceptions in fact are cross-cultural interpretations, rather than the experience of relations with an uncaring provider, what can providers do to correct them? They can pay more attention to what rural people focus on and discuss in everyday life. They also can reflect on *how* people listen to each other. What posture, for example, communicates, "I'm really listening to you"?

Traditions make common discussion topics among rural folk. In healing there are many traditional remedies, of course, and people like to talk about them even if they don't use them anymore. A practitioner who does not indicate an interest in "old-time" cures or folkways is setting up a barrier to communication with the client: "the doctors should respect the home remedies people talk about . . . like lard and soda, or potatoes, or vinegar for burns. But they don't pay any attention to these things [and] patients just don't talk after a while."

Often what the practitioner does talk about is also seen as inappropriate: "Then they ask you all these personal questions . . . about your family and all. . . . You just don't ask people personal questions about their family life. If people want to share something, they'll tell you."

How does the provider get a family history, or a sense of what's going on in a client's life that might be related to a particular problem or set of problems? I'd like to return to the addage "to start where the client is" and refer to Edward T. Hall's concept of high context and low context cultures (in Friedman 1979). Hall argues that most mainstream, urban Americans are low context: we get right down to business. "Efficiency" is a hallmark of our culture; we want to get right down to the matter at hand and, therefore, "tend to put more emphasis on the verbal message and less on the context." Arabs, in contrast, he suggests, are high context in that their communications are set within the context of interpersonal relationships. If you don't take time to establish some sort of relationship with a person, you can't do business with them—unless you do it on the basis of power. Power can come in the form of force, bribes, or bureaucratic role definitions such as case worker and (versus?) client (Friedman 1979; Friedl 1979). But if, like the Arabs, rural folk are high context people, you can be far more effective in relating to them in a context-developing manner.

Local informants suggested how this can be done: "Doctors L and H are just like us. When they come to work, they stop and talk to each one of us. They talk to you like a friend." ("What do you talk about?") "Anything. He'll tell you how his water froze up last night. . . . Just everyday things that we all know . . . the weather, families, feelings."

The doctors indicate by their more high context behavior that people come before business. This mode of relating to people has been described by Herbert Gans as person-orientation as opposed to object-orientation. "Object-oriented individualism involves striving towards the achievement of an 'object.' . . . the overriding aspiration [in person-oriented individualism] is to be a person within the group" (Gans 1962, p. 89).

In applying Gans' concept to rural West Virginians, Weller notes:

You just don't stop in for a moment to check on a detail or two of business, then move on. Each contact is a person-to-person encounter, and this takes time—hours of it. . .

A county school official recently discussed his efforts to see three men who were being chosen for a special training program. It took him six hours because—as he noted—"you can't do business with these people on a time schedule." You must also "set a spell," and in the midst of this person-to-person meeting any business you may have can be done. [Weller 1965, p. 55]

In sum, one gets needed information within the context of a broader social interaction. For the urban-oriented practitioner, it may seem silly to start by talking about the garden or the weather, but that may be the only way ultimately to get down to business. Starting with business invites ineffectiveness. A van driver comments: "When I drive somebody in to the clinic, often he's talked to me for about twenty minutes. . . . Now he doesn't talk with the doctor like that. . . . I could tell the doctor a lot and help make the patient feel more comfortable if he [the doctor] would only listen."

At the Southern Mountain Health Program, rural staff members even map out the correct way a person should come to work in the morning. A well-liked physician stops and talks with each staff member, from the van driver to the receptionist, sometimes taking twenty minutes to get to his own office. By contrast, the "cold" doctor says "hello" to everybody but "he doesn't even break his stride" until he gets to the drug cabinet, which he unlocks before proceeding to patient records and finally to his office. This more object-oriented behavior, so acceptable in an urban context, has caused deep resentment among rural staff and clients, which in turn limits provider effectiveness.

Even physical posture is noticed. The well-accepted physician stands more settled back on his hips, while the "cold doc" leans forward. If the former walked into a wall, his belly would touch first; the latter would have first contact with his forehead. The "belly-first" posture along with other body language such as firmly planted feet and absence of movement, is interpreted as meaning "he really listens to you." The "forehead first" posture on the other hand is somehow disquieting. A walk about the community surrounding the clinic reveals that most men appear to stand in a posture similar to the popular physician. An urban staff member who had moved into the area several years before, and who was a real "forehead man", recalls that a frustrated client had once abruptly told him: "Buddy, I don't even like the way you walk."

Clothing is also symbolic. Rural people often identify denim and old clothes with farm work. I have a farmer for a neighbor who will not come into my house wearing overalls: when he's got farm clothes on, we stand outside and talk; when he's got his slacks and a shirt on, he comes inside. The words of rural staff members in the clinic suggest the attention given to clothing: "I'm tired of apologizing for a doctor who 'looks dirty.' Old clothes say to the client, 'We don't think you're very important.' " "The community asks us what we think about a new doctor. When a new doc comes in, people always call us. . . . They ask, 'Is he clean?' 'Is he hippy looking?' "

It should be noted that cleanliness is associated with certain kinds of clothing. When you are working in and around manure, for example, you wear denim. With the coming of designer jeans, denim has come out of the barnyard a bit, but you may notice that especially when rural women wear them, they have been carefully pressed. Clothing of course can be symbolic of many other things such as wealth, the urban world, and sexuality. It is important to know how clothing is interpreted in a specific community.

In sum, most urban-raised and -trained practitioners are object-oriented people entering a rural, more person-oriented world. How they walk, talk, and dress appears to have an impact upon their effectiveness. It should be noted in passing that there may be a trade-off between effectiveness and individual choice, freedom, and ultimately one's sense of identity as one chooses to conform or not to conform to local norms and patterns of life. One agency director who described himself as "a former hippie" said, "I never feel really comfortable in the clothes I come to work in."

DEFINITIONS OF TIME

In rural life, time is seasonal and natural. There are periods of the year that require fourteen-hour days of intense labor, and there are slack moments when a person can sit back a bit (Campbell 1969). To people brought up in rural environments, the idea that work activity is controlled by a device like a clock seems somewhat artificial. For clients, the idea of punctuality for appointments, which is so deeply imbedded in the value system of health care providers, is taken lightly. In keeping with a person-oriented value system, the appointments record appears to improve with direct contact with the care provider (Friedl 1979).

For rural staff, the idea that a clock rather than work load determines what you can do, seems to be a source of resentment. One clinic secretary confided: "I don't know. I guess I feel watched. Even the director feels he's being watched although I feel he's watching me. I went into his office one day and he was reading *Time* magazine. He looked really embarrassed and dropped the magazine and said, 'It looks like you caught me.' Why can't he realize that I don't care. What's wrong with reading a magazine in a spare moment?" Her statement suggests something else offensive about clocks. They are a behavioral control external to the process of group interaction that is so central and normative in the life of small communities.

PROBLEM SOLVING

Several years ago, an incident at a health services facility in western North Carolina led to a grievance procedure that damaged the agency director's rapport with his staff members. His offense was that he had instructed a van driver to cut the lawn. (The grass had been previously cut by a teenager, who had doubled his rates. The director thought it would be cheaper to buy a lawnmower and give the task to an underutilized van driver. There was no question that the driver had the time to do it.)

To the director, accustomed to the process of decision making through hierarchy, the request seemed routine. To the van driver, who quickly gained the support of the entire rural staff, the request violated a basic rural value of equality and sense of consensus in problem solving. "Why, all he had to say was 'George that grass is gettin' awful high. What do you think we might do about it?' I would have said, 'well, I'll take care of it.'"

As it turned out, the van driver won his grievance. Several hours after the hearing, he mowed the grass without being ordered to do so. And he continued to do it; he had appropriated the job on his own.

A number of students of rural mountain communities emphasize the high value given group solidarity and cohesion at the expense of individual differentiation and achievement. This does not contradict the earlier statements about "Johnny." In a cultural milieu that emphasizes being rather than doing, Johnny *is* still Johnny, the individual. But his individuality is seen within the overall context of the group and interaction based on an ethic of equality and cooperation (Hicks 1976; Matthews 1966). Hierarchical social systems with the vertical lines of authority common to any formal organization such as a mental health clinic stand in sharp contrast to the norms of horizontal relations in group-oriented rural systems. The conflict between vertical and horizontal systems can cause anger, distrust, and refusal to cooperate on the part of both rural clients and staff. A clinic secretary said, "A neighbor of mine said she wouldn't take her medicine unless *I* said it was okay." A van driver reported: "A woman called me last Saturday night and asked if she should take her husband on to the hospital. He was bad off and was supposed to go in on Monday. I asked her if she had called our [doctor on call at the emergency weekend] number. She said, 'No!' She said that she 'could never get anything out of them anyhow' and that she trusted my opinion. So I told her to take him on in. She did."

The rural ethic of equality that underlies an emphasis on horizontal relations requires a kind of cordiality and information sharing foreign to an agency's hierarchal rules of conduct. Some examples: "When somebody comes in [to the clinic] I'm not supposed to [make small] talk to them. But what are they going to think? They're going to say, 'What's happened to her?'" "When a patient asks what his blood pressure is, we aren't supposed to say anything. Then they think something is really wrong. They get scared . . . nervous."

The withholding of information, it should be noted, stratifies an interaction. Those persons having the data control the situation; people without the data are made vulnerable by their ignorance—and they know it. Thus, a potential latent function of hierarchal control of information is feelings of powerlessness and resentment on the part of the client.

Among agency staff, a product of the sense of, as well as the fact of, unequal relations emerges in the feeling that urban professionals don't respect and don't trust their rural coworkers: "He just doesn't seem to trust me. It's funny though, with some things he does . . . all that money coming in and I account for it. He trusts me with the books . . . but not with the key to the office." "He trusts me in my job, but not as a person . . . I can't just talk to [the agency director]. I have to follow the chain of command." "They're always checking on us." "Why don't they trust us?"

Obviously, these feelings complicate an agency's operation and effectiveness. The hierarchical approach to problem solving and task completion is often dysfunctional in the rural setting, requiring special sensitivity and creativity on the part of supervisory staff.

IS CHANGE "PROGRESS"?

A woman who recently moved to a rural community expressed frustration over the fact that local women on an agency staff seemed to isolate her in the work environment. One of the local women responded: "Well, I guess your little boy is just about the same age as mine. Every Sunday we walk down the road together and to church just like I did when I was a little girl. And when he grows up, I want him to be walking down that road to that church. But you . . . you . . . people like you come in here and change everything. And I don't want things to change. I don't want change . . . I want things to stay as they are."

Change has been defined as progress, by an urbanizing, industrializing America since the mid-nineteenth century. In mainstream culture, progress is such a deeply imbued value that to oppose it is something akin to subversion. And yet, the history of change, in rural Appalachia at least, is one of the destruction of family and community life, of the impoverishment of a region and its people (Eller 1982; Gaventa 1980). So history has taught many people in Appalachia to fear change. Additionally, at the cultural level, agricultural societies tend to value balance and a cyclical sense of renewal over linear change (Diamond 1974). The value conflict between balance and progress is a source of client and staff anxiety, rooted in both historical reality and cultural norms. Urban staff members might do well to look at their own assumptions about "progress" and the notion that change always means improvement.

THE SACRED IN EVERYDAY LIFE

If people define a situation as real, it is real in its consequences (Thomas 1978). God is real and Christ as God Incarnate is real to many people. They are significant others to whom some rural Appalachians turn in discerning what is right and what ought to be done (Coles 1971). I asked Southern Mountain Health Program staff members, "What persons or figures do you think of as being important to you in the evaluation of your actions?" The professionals uniformly answer "family, friends, and peers." Several rural staff members started their lists of significant others with "God." If God is a concrete, personal experience, His impact on individual identity, one's sense of purpose in life and crises, can be enormous. Practitioners counseling rural clients know the power of the sacred in healing; time and again clients tell of terrible experiences that have made them wonder how they could continue to function at all. The answers to inquiries into the source of a client's strength seem remarkably consistent: "I know God loves me;" "Jesus is always there;" "He gives me strength;" "He was teaching me."

The practitioner born and trained in a secular urban world is ill equipped to deal with or reinforce such testimony even when it is efficacious in treatment. Mental health providers who can respond become sought after as "Christian counselors," although most of them eschew the label.

If the world of the sacred in the southern mountains includes the Christian God and His Son Incarnate, it also includes the Devil and Hell for many people. A therapist reported the following hallucinatory

episode that occurred in the midst of a counseling session: "I'm falling. . . . See the Devil there [pointing to another family member pres-
ent] . . . he say's I'm falling into Hell . . . I can see the flame. . . . Oh,
please help me. . . ." ("Can you see your feet?") "Yes." ("Can you
see your feet on the floor?") "Yes." ("Can you see my feet on the
floor?") "Yes." ("Then you're not falling. You know the Devil is a
liar. Everybody knows that. You can see all our feet, all our feet on
the floor. Everybody knows the Devil is a liar.") The episode was
eased to the point where the patient was able to take part in the
development of a treatment plan.

CULTURAL ILLITERACY AMONG PROVIDERS

Participating in this sort of dialogue can be unsettling for any provider;
but for those raised and trained in a cultural milieu that ignores or
denies sacred definitions of the world, the interaction becomes especially foreign and uncomfortable. (This was demonstrated at a recent workshop, where I gave this as a case study to clinical social
workers and asked them how they would have handled it.) Appropriate training could make this aspect of mountain culture more familiar and comprehensible to practitioners coming into the area,
ameliorating their discomfort and enabling them to better serve their
clients. Training should also help the provider understand the eth-
nocentricism arising out of his or her own background that may block
the ability to empathize with the patient. Two recommendations of
Spector's analysis of cultural diversity in health and illness are especially appropriate here: ethnic studies must be taken by all people
who wish to deliver health care; and the health care provider must
be sensitive to his own perceptions of health and illness and practices
he employs (Spector 1979, p. 293).

The ethnocentrism that has not understood the need for ethnic
studies has also not seen the need for the kind of research that would
yield the data needed for such studies. For example, a psychiatrist
recently told me he notices a significant difference in symptoms between his rural Appalachian patients and those in a previous practice
in the Middle West. "I had read about hysterical conversion," he says,
"but you just didn't see it out there. There seems to be a lot of it
here." He also reports seeing much visual hallucination. Having
worked with cancer patients who report having "visions," which they
themselves thought might be a side effect of pain medication, I wonder about the role of "cultural permission" in mental illness. Do fun-

damentalist religious views perhaps legitimate certain symptomatic responses in rural Appalachia? Are hallucinations OK if they are defined as "visions"? In sum, do Appalachians and Americans from other regions get "sick" in different ways? What is the role of Appalachian culture in sickness and health? More research is needed.

This study of a primary health care delivery system and of mental health delivery in a western North Carolina Appalachian county finds significant differences in the interpretation of behavior and symbols between local Appalachian staff members and nonlocal in-migrant providers, raised and trained in urban mainstream American culture. The differences proved damaging to the health care delivery process. The success of the encounter session between local and in-migrant staff members demonstrates the need for training for providers in local world views, values, and behavior. The need for training, in turn, underlines the need for more research on cultural differences in the Appalachian region.

REFERENCES

Campbell, J.C. 1969. *The southern highlander and his homeland*. Lexington: University Press of Kentucky (originally published 1921).

Carlisle, R., and D. Monteith. 1983. *Economic development: Trends and implications for western North Carolina*. Cullowhee: Western North Carolina Tomorrow.

Coles, R. 1971. *Children of crisis*, vol. 2, *Migrants, sharecroppers, mountaineers*. Boston: Little, Brown.

Diamond, S. 1974. *In search of the primitive, a critique of civilization*. New Brunswick, N.J.: Transaction Books.

Duran, R. 1975. *Chicano plan for mental health*. Springfield, Va.: National Technical Information Service.

Eller, R.D. 1982. *Miner, millhands and mountaineers: Industrialization of the Appalachian south, 1880-1930*. Knoxville: University of Tennessee Press.

Friedl, J. 1979. Appalachian stereotypes and their impact on health care. Paper presented at the 78th Annual Meeting of the American Anthropological Association, Cincinnati.

Friedman, K. 1979. Learning the Arab's silent language. An interview with Edward T. Hall. *Psychology Today* 13(3): 45-54.

Gans, H. 1962. *The urban villagers*. New York: Free Press.

Gaventa, J. 1980. *Power and powerlessness: Quiescence and rebellion in an Appalachian valley*. Urbana: University of Illinois Press.

Glasscote, R., D. Sanders, H.M. Forstenzer, and A.R. Foley. 1964. *The community mental health center. An analysis of existing models*. Washington, D.C.: Joint Information Service of the American Psychiatric Association and the National Association for Mental Health.

Hicks, G. 1976. *Appalachian valley*. New York: Holt, Rinehart & Winston.

Houpt, J.L., C.S. Orleans, L.K. George, and H.K.H. Brodie. 1979. *The importance of mental health services to general health care*. Cambridge, Mass.: Ballinger.

Keefe, S.E., and J.M. Casas. 1980. Mexican Americans and mental health: A selected review and recommendations for mental health service delivery. *American Journal of Community Psychology* 8:303-26.

Knight, J.A., and W.E. Davis. 1969. *Manual for the comprehensive community mental health clinic*. Englewood Cliffs, N.J.: Prentice-Hall.

Lewis, H. 1971. Medicos and mountaineers: The meeting of two cultures. Banquet speech given at the Appalachian Regional Hospital's Spring Scientific Session, Asheville, N.C.

Matthews, E.M. 1966. *Neighbor and kin: Life in a Tennessee ridge community*. Nashville: Vanderbilt University.

Mechanic, D. 1979. *Mental health and social policy*. Englewood Cliffs, N.J.: Prentice Hall.

Spector, R.E. 1979. *Cultural diversity in health and illness*. New York: Appleton-Century-Crofts.

Thomas, C.S., and J.P. Comer. 1973. Racism and mental health services. In *Racism and mental health*, eds. C.W. Willie, B.M. Kramer, and B.S. Brown. Pittsburgh: University of Pittsburgh Press.

Thomas, W.I. 1978. The definition of the situation. In *Symbolic interaction: A reader in social psychology*, eds. J.G. Manis & B.N. Meltzer. 3d ed. Boston: Allyn & Bacon.

Torrey, E.F. 1970. The irrelevancy of traditional mental health services for urban Mexican-Americans. *American Journal of Orthopsychiatry* 40:240-41.

Weller, J.E. 1965. *Yesterday's people: Life in contemporary Appalachia*. Lexington: University Press of Kentucky.

12

Appalachian Family Therapy

CYNTHIA COLE

There has been a growing interest among therapists in considering the cultural context when practicing family therapy (McGoldrick, Pearce, and Giordano 1982). During the early 1960s, several family therapists found that a given intervention approach was more or less effective depending on a family's socioeconomic status (Hoffman 1981). This realization led to the development of several different "schools" of therapy that took into account the ecological setting in which the family was embedded. Gradually, the notion of ecological setting was refined to include not only income level and education but also ethnicity (Haley 1973).

Although there is at least minimal information available concerning several American cultural groups, little has been written concerning the process of family therapy with the Appalachian family. To fill some of this gap, Mountain Youth Resources, a private, nonprofit social work agency providing family therapy in the western counties of North Carolina, has developed a summary of Appalachian family characteristics to assist in planning family interventions. This paper describes the agency, basic family systems concepts, the therapy process, relevant Appalachian characteristics, and an example of work with a composite family drawn from several real cases. The summary of characteristics has been based primarily on observation and experience with mountain families and secondarily on inferences from other written observations of Appalachian culture (Caudill 1962; Reul 1974; Weller 1965).

MOUNTAIN YOUTH RESOURCES

Mountain Youth Resources (MYR) was founded in 1979 as part of the move to develop community-based alternatives to juvenile incarceration. The agency emphasizes early intervention and works to keep referred youth with their families and to use community resources to strengthen the family unit. MYR offers home-based family therapy,

development of community aid, and a temporary group-home shelter
to youths (ages 10-17) and their families in Cherokee, Swain, Jackson,
and Haywood Counties. Families are referred to MYR by schools,
courts, social services, and others when adolescents experience trouble at home, in school, or in the community.

Suspected child abuse or neglect; truant, withdrawn, or illegal child
behavior; and poor school performance might cause an agency or
individual to make an MYR referral. Most parents of troubled children
have a desire to improve their difficult home situation, and MYR
draws upon that to assist the family in working together to resolve
their problems. Often this achieves MYR's goal of strengthening the
family unit, which in turn supports individual growth for all members.
Though MYR believes that the family is the best place for a child to
receive support and guidance, it is useful at times to give a troubled
family a breather. Hawthorne House provides up to ninety days of
care for youth who require it while the family work goes on.

FAMILY SYSTEMS THERAPY

Over the past twenty years, the emerging field of family therapy has
developed several widely accepted concepts that form the basis for
the approach in any cultural setting. The most fundamental concept
is that each member affects and is affected by every other member.
These relationships form an interlocking network, such that a stress
at one point of the family system causes a reaction at other points.
Unspoken marital conflict thus may result not in open hostility between the parents but in the couple's adolescent son running away
from home. A therapeutic response to the situation must take into
account the meaning of the individual's behavior in the family context.
The family therapist sees the family as the locus of the problem and
the locus of the solution.

Families have intricate mechanisms for adapting to change and yet
maintaining stability over time (Carter and McGoldrick 1980). Families with fewer adaptive resources tend to be more rigidly organized
or more chaotic than families with a greater range of successful behaviors. Family therapy attempts to strengthen the marital (or executive) subsystem, increase behavioral options for individuals and the
group, and support individuals in defining who they want to be and
can be, while maintaining family ties and support. Several possible
approaches to achieving these goals include parental education, marital therapy, assertiveness and communication training for adoles-

cents, job skills training to enable youth to leave home appropriately, and assisting the family to improve finances, housing, or community support.

APPALACHIAN FAMILY CHARACTERISTICS

To apply the general concepts of family therapy to a particular family, the therapist must consider the impact of a broader system: the family's sociocultural milieu. Effective therapy in Harlem is not the same as effective therapy in Bryson City, North Carolina. Even so, although some general cultural themes are expressed among Appalachians or blacks or other ethnic groups, cultures change, traditional groups become modern, and each family creates its unique reality, just as surely as mountains create their own weather within the context of overall weather conditions. With this in mind, the MYR therapists use the general Appalachian family characteristics to begin exploration of the ways in which a given family fits or does not fit the expected picture.

In general, these characteristics are found more often among families who have lived in the region for several generations. Limited contact with other cultural options, whether from financial, educational, or geographic immobility, also is associated with families that demonstrate the Appalachian characteristics described. The following description thus applies more often and more accurately to geographically isolated, rural, and possibly, poor families.

For the therapist, who may well be from outside the region, the first characteristic to cause a direct impact is an Appalachian tendency to view outsiders with reservation or suspicion. The attitude is well founded as outsiders have frequently been deliberately exploitive (Beaver, Chapter 1; Caudill 1962). More subtle in their detrimental effects have been groups of "helpers," some of whom have represented different but powerful social and value systems, against which the mountain culture has had difficulty asserting itself (Beaver, Chapter 1; Weller 1965). These experiences make MYR help less available or appealing to some families. It thus becomes essential to establish the therapist's acceptance of and respect for family hierarchy and customs at the initial contact.

Related to this are the Appalachian values of personal autonomy and family self-sufficiency. The male mountaineer historically was his own provider, law, and protector, his family's agent to the outside world, and teacher to his children. The family functioned independently both economically and socially. Family strength was enhanced by the effort to "help our own" but flexibility was diminished by attempting to meet most needs within the family. For some families, this tendency even contributed to weakening the incest taboo. Overall, mountain families have been relatively closed systems, which implies some difficulties getting information and services across their boundaries. Some families do not participate readily in community service programs or classes. Even community institutions like schools, medical facilities, and the police may be regarded with suspicion and hostility. Mountain people respond more favorably to individuals than agencies and are unimpressed by professional hierarchy. Social agencies like mental health, welfare, and family services are especially suspect because families are expected to care for their own members. An "outsider" should "leave well enough alone."

For all these reasons, outreach mental health programs are often more effective in rural Appalachia than the more usual clinic-based programs. The increased cost of individual therapists going into the community to work with families is offset by increased effectiveness. Within those family system boundaries, there is often a large and complex network of subsystems and roles constrained to a small geographic, emotional, and social space. One MYR client estimated that he had 67 relatives living within one hollow. The mental health worker looking for a nuclear family in which to intervene often feels confused and helpless, along with the urge to ask, "Will this child's real mother please stand up?"

Men and women tend to have well-defined roles and rather separate lives, with the men managing life outside the home and the women managing life inside. Both men and women maintain control over their spheres by withholding details about activities. Not as carefully defined are generational boundaries and narrow definitions of mother and father. Many family members participate in child rearing, which can provide many additional resources as well as some confusion about responsibility when things go awry.

Though family size is diminishing as more women are employed outside the home, children are still highly valued and give meaning to their parents' lives. Mothers will often say their children come before everything else. Even though physical discipline is sometimes harsh, as parents attempt to build "character," child rearing is generally permissive and focuses on what pleases the child. Mothers, especially, may feel unable or unwilling to control children who are difficult to manage, and both parents may feel their job is finished when the child is thirteen or fourteen years of age.

Appalachian families have deep psychological ties to their mountains. Reul (1974) has noted that these ties are focused on their "homeplace," the ancestral home or location where their families have lived for generations. This is not necessarily viewed as a place of beauty but as "my place, where I belong and which I control" (Reul 1974, p. 235). Reul also states, "there is a mountain expression that a child should never move further away than you could see the smoke from his chimney" (1974, p. 239). This saying expresses well the intensity of the tie to home and family often felt by Appalachians.

This tie also is the source of a firmly held commitment to help kin whether or not one likes them or has the emotional and financial resources at hand to do so. Many families will stretch their resources beyond the breaking point before resorting to outside help for overwhelming adversities. By the time a family therapist is involved, the family has undergone tremendous suffering and may have lost a good deal of its structural cohesiveness.

Reul states that "the mountain family is a closely knit one, not primarily because of shared activities but because of emotional dependence. Early childhood training and experience not only foster loyalty to the family but encourage emotional dependence upon the parents" (Reul 1974, p. 242). This dependence contributes to conformity and control of their own behavior. Expansiveness of any kind—whether it be emotional expression, physical movement, or allowing themselves or their children to take up "breathing room" in the world—is discouraged. For the therapist primarily trained to "talk out feelings," this presents quite a challenge because a very different set of therapeutic skills is required.

Because the Appalachian will often value family loyalty above making it in the outside world, there is somewhat less voluntary migration out of their communities. Families prefer to stay nearby even though greater economic opportunity exists elsewhere. School achievement may not be valued highly if it interferes with family activities or responsibilities and politics and social systems tend to be based on a "family loyalty" rather than a "fairness" standard. Each generation may have an explorer or two who migrates out into the world, but they later tend to move back home. During economic hard times, when mountain people have been forced to leave, it has caused great emotional pain.

This tie to the land is also the most frequent source of conflict with the value of family loyalty. It appears that more family disputes result from boundary line disagreements and the need to split up the "home place" than any other single event in Appalachian culture. Family members carry memories for generations concerning how relatives received parcels of land that should have been theirs or how land was sold out of the family to "foreigners"—either unrelated families or, worse, people from out of state.

Religion in Appalachia is also the source of strongly held family beliefs. Doctrines that emphasize the evil and powerlessness of man are firmly rooted. In addition, religious beliefs are pervasive, even for those who don't attend church, and encourage endurance, acceptance of the Lord's will, and an absence of personal responsibility and initiative concerning the events or circumstances of one's life. Family members thus rarely believe they can or should deliberately have an impact on the world, yet they are deeply offended by individuals or institutions that don't treat them respectfully. It's not "their place" to tell someone else how to behave, but they certainly know how they and others "should" behave. For the family therapist, these attitudes make interventions based on "taking charge of your life" difficult or impossible.

Another belief that tends to isolate the individual or family from seeking outside help is reflected in the sayings: "The Lord won't put any more on you than you can handle," "We have to take what the Lord sends us," and "He knows best." The mountaineer usually interprets these to mean that the solutions to life's difficulties must come from within and from spiritual beliefs. In light of these strongly held values and beliefs, some therapists have become students of the Bible to muster additional, culturally esteemed support for their recommendations.

These characteristics of Appalachian families, while not universal, are common enough that the family therapist working in the region is well-advised to keep them in mind. Families who have been in the region for generations and who have been isolated tend to exhibit them to one degree or another. Effective therapy requires working within the value system and cultural orientation of the families served by the therapist. Application of these concepts to a case example will clarify these points.

THE BUCKNER FAMILY

The case chosen to illustrate the Appalachian family problems with which Mountain Youth Resources deals is a composite of several different families. The details have been changed to protect the families involved, but the issues and conflicts described are representative and

Figure 12.1. Genogram of the Buckner Family

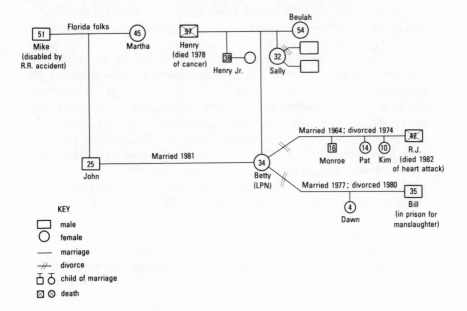

KEY

☐ male
◯ female
── marriage
⫲ divorce
☖ ☗ child of marriage
⊠ ⊗ death

common. Each generation in this family holds a different combination of traditional and modern values, generating significant family stress.

The basic structure of the family is diagrammed in the family genogram (Figure 12.1). The genogram is a family tree on which can be recorded social, physical, and demographic information. It is an essential tool for the family therapist, who must have a picture of family members, their relationships, significant stresses and change points, conflicts, strengths, and other information.

The Buckner family was referred to MYR by social services following an abuse complaint. The complaint stated that John Buckner had beaten his four-old stepdaughter. In addition, his sixteen-old stepson was reported as being "disrespectful" to John when the stepson attempted to discipline his younger siblings. After an investigation, social services determined that a beating had not occurred but an excessive spanking had. While the situation did not involve actual abuse or neglect, the social service worker felt that the family would benefit a great deal from family therapy.

While initiating the family treatment, the MYR therapist gathered data on individual family members and family dynamics. The nuclear family unit consists of John and Betty Buckner and Betty's four children from two previous marriages. John and Betty, married for two years, state that they love each other and want their relationship to work, but that they are experiencing some difficulty. The marriage is John's first and Betty's third.

John, who is nine years younger than Betty, moved to North Carolina with his family six years ago, after his father was disabled. He graduated from high school and has been working as an orderly at the same hospital where Betty works. As an only child, he is unfamiliar with the pressures and "interference" of a large family network. He also has poor impulse control under stress. With little experience, he is attempting to play out his idea of paterfamilias in a system that finds him wanting on many counts: his age, his "foreign" status, and his lack of skills and background for the task he has undertaken.

Betty comes to the marriage with four children and two failed marriages behind her. An intelligent woman, her year of "advanced training" enabling her to work as an LPN sets her apart from her family. Her previous life choices indicate that she has wavered between traditional and modern Appalachian values throughout her adult life. Her initial marital choice was a traditional one, but her second marriage to an American Indian was based on her wish to establish her independence from her family. Her choice of John appears to represent the following for Betty: (1) a wish to "fit in" to her family system by the choice of a spouse who is closer to her family's requirements than her second husband; (2) a continuing disregard for family pressure to marry within the cultural group; (3) the first time her marital choice would permit her to establish equal power in the relationship, since she selected a younger, less experienced man. Her extreme passivity in previous marriages plus her present choice of a man with so much less power than hers are patterns associated with women who have been physically or sexually abused as children. This possibility has not yet been substantiated, however.

The oldest child, Monroe, had a good though distant relationship with his father, R.J., whom he saw only occasionally after his parents' divorce until R.J.'s death. Monroe's relationship with Bill, Betty's second husband, was strained because Bill was violent with Betty and Monroe felt protective of her. After Bill went to jail, Monroe stepped even further into the "parental child" role, assuming quite a bit of responsibility for his sisters, including discipline. This role, though difficult for someone his age, provided him with status in the family and, from the beginning of the marriage, he has been suspicious of

John's efforts to take over the role. When John began to have difficulty with Dawn, the youngest child, culminating in the excessive spanking that resulted in the DSS referral, Monroe became overtly hostile toward John. They have not dealt openly with the conflict, but Monroe now challenges John whenever he attempts to discipline the girls in any way. Monroe also seems confused by the fact that his mother, Betty, alternates between support for Monroe and support for John, as each plays "father" to the younger children.

Beulah, Betty's mother, who lives nearby, is not ambivalent about her support, however. She has clearly aligned herself with Monroe whom, at sixteen, she sees as the "man of the family." He is the true Appalachian and she feels strongly that she doesn't want her grandchildren raised by an outsider. Since her husband, Henry, died in 1978, she has been more involved with all of her children. As a wife, Beulah was overtly submissive, but controlled her husband through manipulation. Beulah tolerated Betty's first husband because he was a hometown boy, but despised the second because he is Indian, domineering, and violent. She simply does not value John because he is a Floridian, too young, and in her opinion not good enough for Betty.

For the first time, both Beulah and Betty have a man in the family system who is not clearly dominant. This presents opportunities and terrors for each of them that their Appalachian culture has not provided guidelines for handling. Since the man in question is also an outsider trying to fit into an indigenous family system, there is an overt level of hostility and rejection by Beulah and Monroe, the two most committed to standing for traditional values. Beulah has formed a coalition with her grandson across generational boundaries that is undermining John and Betty's attempts to form a well-functioning parental subsystem.

Because of their different cultural backgrounds, John and Betty have different perspectives about what level of involvement in the Buckner family is appropriate for Beulah. Betty is attempting to form a modern egalitarian marriage within a context of personal passivity and cultural support for male dominance. Her choice of John is an attempt to balance power in the marital relationship, but she also has a cultural blind spot that prevents her from seeing clearly how her mother's coalition with Monroe interferes. She is much more accustomed than John to extended family participation in nuclear family affairs and cannot pinpoint this as a problem. John, on his part, does *not* expect such involvement and resents his wife's wavering between support for him and support for her mother. His feeling of being an outsider leads him to redouble his efforts to establish his authority over the children. This leads Monroe and Beulah to redouble their efforts to discount and undermine John, causing him to feel rejected and even more of an outsider in an endless, escalating behavioral cycle.

The Mountain Youth Resources social worker assigned to the family thus finds them caught in a runaway feedback system, where each solution attempted becomes part of the problem, intensifying the original difficulty. This sequence is repeated over and over with the family becoming more distressed each time. To break into this destructive loop, the therapist works with the family to attempt the following:

1. Rebalance the system so that each member feels valued for an appropriate role. Thus, children are children, parents are parents, extended family are valued advisors but not active participants within the family.

2. Assist John in finding a personal niche within this Appalachian family to reduce his feeling of being an outsider.

3. Strengthen the marital-parental subsystem of John and Betty to meet their goal of establishing an egalitarian marriage.

4. Provide both Beulah and Monroe with roles of authority as holders of Appalachian lore that support not undermine John and Betty's executive role.

5. Provide John with specific training in effective parenting to increase his skills to match those of other family members.

Just as the characteristics of Appalachian families must be considered to understand the development of this family's difficulties, the plan for meeting these goals must also consider the same issues. The plan calls for less talking and more action than might be appropriate with other cultural groups. The plan also uses ideas and activities that are already familiar to and valued by this family. Asking the family to conceptualize the problem as the therapist does is not as important as direct suggestions, which in themselves bring about the rebalancing desired.

The plan includes the following suggestions:

1. John, who knows little about hunting and fishing, is to ask Monroe, who knows a great deal, to go on periodic trips including these activities. This accomplishes several things. By increasing John's

understanding of and skills in traditional Appalachian activities, his ability to establish a niche improves. Monroe can take a position of authority in this area, which may make it easier for him to give up the authority over the children's discipline, leaving that to John and Betty.

2. Monroe is to be encouraged to hunt and fish for the family and to cut and stack the wood. This also acknowledges a developing adult role in the family.

3. John is to seek out Beulah's views on child rearing and perhaps to raise a garden with her. This also has several purposes. It enables Beulah to pass on valuable information to John, but allows him to control how he uses it. It enables John and Beulah to have a direct relationship, rather than going through Betty. It also tends to remove Beulah from her coalition with Monroe on child rearing issues. Like Monroe, Beulah wants a viable role in the family. As a valued Appalachian culture and child-care expert, she may be willing to give up her more disruptive activities.

4. Both John and Betty are to share their family history and traditions with a special eye for differences. This will enable them to clarify how they want to manage roles and expectations.

5. Betty and John are to take the STEP program (Systematic Training for Effective Parenting) together. This will fill in some of John's experience gaps and equalize their power around parenting issues. It points out to the family system that they are to be the parents and provides them with much needed skills development.

With these recommendations, this family may be able to reduce the areas of conflict that are making it difficult for them to meet family responsibilities for child rearing. Their main difficulties revolve around three issues: the changing nature of the modern world, which requires a change in the roles of men and women; the difference in values from one generation to the next, caused in part by the first issue; and the challenge of incorporating a "stranger" into the family. The plan is designed to modify the structure of the family sufficiently to enable the family to resolve these issues.

This case description illustrates how a therapist can use an understanding of Appalachian culture within the broad context of family therapy. The main goal of the family therapist in any culture is to function within the family and community value system sufficiently that the recommendations can be assimilated while shifting or reframing behaviors that have become dysfunctional. It is a concept widely held in family therapy, for example, that the executive or parental subsystem must have enough autonomy to provide an authoritative structure that facilitates child rearing. Yet, this general principle must be applied to the Appalachian family while still acknowledging and honoring the family's membership in the distinctive Appalachian culture that values family ties across generations. There is wide variation among American subcultures concerning how much cross-generational involvement among adult family members is appropriate. One example is the stereotyped Jewish mother, who has become a symbol of overinvolvement with adult children. In contrast, the Irish mother may not speak to a grown child for long periods of time without considering it inappropriate.

The therapist must recognize that cultures have evolved mechanisms for ensuring both stability and adaptability just as families and individuals have done so. The customs that result from the culture's best attempt to resolve environmental challenge should command respect and loyalty, even after the original challenge has passed out of memory. In evaluating the Jewish and Irish solutions to the role of mother, which represent opposite ends of the involvement continuum, it is essential to recognize that at one time each of those responses was an effective solution to a real problem. The loyalty to custom is reasonably based on that fact, even though that same custom may have become dysfunctional in current applications.

The Appalachian culture offers many potent resources for the therapist willing to work within a cultural framework. The therapist working against cultural forces may well find those same potent forces marshaled against change perceived as too fast or too destructive of deeply held family values.

NOTES

I would like to thank Jim Anderson, Harry Manes, Peter Ray, and Charles Ryer who were members of the Mountain Youth Resources staff at the time this paper was written and contributed to the paper's conceptualization.

REFERENCES

Caudill, H.M. 1962. *Night comes to the Cumberlands*. Boston: Little, Brown.
Carter, B., and M. McGoldrick. 1980. *The family life cycle*. New York: Gardner Press.
Haley, J. 1973. *Uncommon therapy*. New York: W.W. Norton & Co.
Hoffman, L. 1981. *Foundations of family therapy*. New York: Basic Books.

McGoldrick, M., J. Pearce, and J. Giordano. 1982. *Ethnicity and family therapy*. New York: The Guilford Press.

Reul, M.R. 1974. *Territorial boundaries of rural poverty*. East Lansing: Center for Rural Manpower and Public Affairs and the Cooperative Extension Service, Michigan State University.

Weller, J.E. 1965. *Yesterday's people*. Lexington: University Press of Kentucky.

13

Hospitalized Appalachian Adolescents

RHODA H. HALPERIN AND MARCIA SLOMOWITZ

One morning, early, my mother took me to her and told me she needed me to stay home and be at her side. I was happy. I said I was glad to do anything she wanted. She held me close and said thanks. I remember feeling really good the rest of the day. But at night, in bed, I felt sad and my eyes became all filled up, and I didn't know why. [Coles and Coles 1978, p. 77]

This paper focuses upon relationships among rural to urban migration patterns, changing gender roles, and transformations in family structure as factors that place urban Appalachian adolescents at risk for serious psychiatric disorders. A number of transitions, rooted in economic, life course, and institutional processes, affect the mental health of rural Appalachian migrants in cities. These include change in physical environment, adaptation to an urban versus rural way of life, change in dependence upon subsistence production to reliance upon wage labor, and change in social networks. Typically, the literature describes the impact of rural to urban migration on economic, psychological, and social outcomes for the individual, group (family), and receiving community (Schwarzweller and Brown 1970; Schwarzweller, Brown, and Mangalam 1971). With the exception of the work of Looff (1971; Looff and Smith 1969) and Coles (1971), the persons depicted in the family are the adults.[1] Because adolescent children of adult migrants face an additional transition, as they are in a transitional stage in the life course, they experience rural-urban culture change differently from adults. Many experience both transitions quite acutely, with decreasing ability to function well; in extreme cases some require psychiatric hospitalization for severe psychological distress.

Our data are selected from the adolescent psychiatry inpatient service of an urban university teaching hospital adjacent to an Appalachian region. The city of Cincinnati has long received Appalachian migrants from counties in eastern Kentucky, West Virginia, and Tennessee, as well as from rural Ohio. Most of the adolescents on the service are from lower socioeconomic classes. In all families, one or both parents may be unemployed or employed at a subsistence wage. The family system often is dysfunctional in its present environment. Of the approximately 135 adolescents between the ages of thirteen and seventeen hospitalized on the service each year, about 20 percent are Appalachian in the sense that their families originated in rural Ohio, Kentucky, Tennessee, or West Virginia.[2] The average length of stay in the hospital is one month. The clinical impression is that the spectrum of clinical diagnoses in Appalachian adolescents admitted to the unit is no different from the spectrum of diagnoses for non-Appalachian patients.[3] The range of psychiatric disorders and problems seen in the hospital includes depression with suicidal thought or behavior, behavioral problems, often with associated refusal and/or avoidance of school, legal difficulties, and drug and alcohol abuse. Few have psychotic illnesses, such as schizophrenia or bipolar affective disorder. These disorders tend to manifest themselves later in life.

As such, then, the presenting symptoms of Appalachian adolescents appear to be no different from those of other adolescents on the unit. All of the adolescents require hospitalization because of multiple problems, such as depression, behavioral problems, severe family discord, substance abuse, suicidal ideation, and psychotic disorders. The specific social context varies among the Appalachian adolescents, and it is important to understand the nature of the urban experience for people who differ in rural adaptations, for example, rural farms versus rural coal mining regions with dependency upon wage labor. Understanding the specific meaning of the homeplace and its implications, both psychological and economic, is also critical. The residence pattern, furthermore, is a distinctive one of bilocal residence (frequent and patterned movements of both adolescents and their families back and forth between urban dwellings and the rural homeplace). These elements of the Appalachian migrants' experience must be taken into account in order to understand their behavior as adaptive or maladaptive.

We focus upon two detailed case analyses of hospitalized Appalachian adolescents. Both patients are young women from rural Appalachian backgrounds. These particular cases highlight mental health issues and adjustment problems as well as issues of generation, gender, and class. Both adolescents are first-generation urban residents from poor families, who were part of the most recent wave of rural to urban migration (McCoy and Brown 1981; Philliber and McCoy

1981; Schwarzweller and Brown 1970). These two patients have typical problems (Danna 1980; Brody 1970). They do not represent extremes in any sense; the patients are not delinquents, chronic substance abusers, criminals, or violent individuals. Neither patient is psychotic; and neither has a major mental disorder, such as schizophrenia or bipolar affective disorder. No doubt a parallel analysis could be done with men patients. We chose two women to highlight patterns of behavior between parents and children and to draw contrasts between rural agrarian and rural wage labor backgrounds. By eliminating the variable of sex, we can draw a more controlled and systematic comparison.

Our analysis uses the collaborative experience of the service's attending psychiatrist, the nurses, social workers, and the psychiatry department's anthropologist. The analysis derives from discussions in treatment team meetings and teaching sessions on the adolescent inpatient service.

Our central hypothesis is that interrelated economic, social and psychological conditions, in which the pattern of bilocal residence (involving back and forth movements from the urban environment to the rural homeplace) figures importantly, place the two patients in the untenable role of culture broker. Their broker roles are exaggerated by their mothers' sense of powerlessness. By anthropological definition, culture brokers are mediators between two cultures: here, rural and urban. In order to play the role effectively individuals must command economic resources, possess political sophistication, and be able to switch appropriately in and out of the two cultures. As Eric Wolf defines it, the position of culture broker "is an 'exposed' one, since, Janus-like, they face in two directions at once. They must serve some of the interests of groups operating on both the community and national level, and they must cope with the conflict raised by the collision of these interests" (Wolf 1956, p. 1076). Unfortunately, in the adolescent phase of life, broker roles are not viable psychologically, economically, or behaviorally, because the role places too many conflicting demands upon the youths. They have neither the psychological security, the economic resources, nor the social skills to meet the demands. They find it difficult to adapt simultaneously to dual environments, rural and urban; because their identities are unformed, they cannot easily switch back and forth from rural to urban roles. The multiple conflicts can become too great for the adolescents to manage, and they can become severely maladapted: they "fit" neither in rural nor in urban cultures. Serious symptoms requiring hospitalization can subsequently emerge.

Although we cannot address the questions of why some adolescents manage both the life course and the geographic transitions better than others or why some adolescents require hospitalization and others do not, we think these are critical issues raised by the two cases. We examine the role of two adolescent women as culture brokers and the conditions under which the role is developed, sustained, and ultimately changed in the therapeutic process. We pay particular attention to the adaptation problems (economic, cultural, and psychological) of the adolescents' mothers, since their problems contribute to their daughters' disorders. Since the patients and their mothers make repeated visits to their rural places of origin, in effect becoming biresidential, the importance of homeplace ties becomes poignantly evident in both cases.

Adolescence is the time when the individual develops a sense of self as both a member of one's own family, and as a future developer of another family. From a psychological perspective, the primary task of adolescence is the development of an identity. Since the publication of Margaret Mead's book, *Coming of Age in Samoa* (1928), the treatment of adolescence as a life phase, from both a psychiatric and an anthropological perspective, has attracted considerable attention. Recently, the work of Offer and Peterson (Offer, Ostrov, and Howard 1981; Peterson and Offer 1979) has shown normal American adolescence also to be a relatively smooth time. It is a time of transition, of social and psychological change for individuals, but it is normally not a time of turmoil. When there is turmoil, anguish, and extreme discord within the family, that is a sign of abnormality. Hospitalization on an inpatient psychiatric unit indicates distress severe enough such that the individual cannot be maintained in the family and the community. In the hospital context, issues of family structure, problems of adaptation to urban environments, and conflicts between rural and urban systems of expectations become apparent in the presenting symptoms of adolescents and in the subsequent management of the illness problems. The paper now turns to the adolescents under discussion.

TERESA

Teresa is a sixteen-year-old Caucasian adolescent. She was hospitalized for six weeks. Her presenting symptoms included a two-month history of depression with irritability, a ten-pound weight loss, reduced involvement in usual activities, sometimes staying in bed, and alcohol abuse with binges on weekends. One month prior to admission, she took a drug overdose. Six months prior to admission, she dropped out of school. Teresa and her family were seen intermittently by a social worker in their community when in crisis.

*Family History.*Teresa is one of six children. She has a sister, age nineteen, unmarried, who lives out of the home with her two-year-old child and has a drug problem; a brother, seventeen, with alcoholism; a fourteen-year-old brother; and a ten-year-old brother, noted by the community social worker to have school phobia. Teresa lives with her mother, who has been divorced for seven years. Her father, an alcoholic, lives in Florida.

Teresa's mother migrated from her family's farm in Tennessee to Cincinnati because she saw the move as a source of economic opportunity. Although Teresa's mother readily sought jobs, she kept no job longer than a few months. At the time of Teresa's admission, her mother worked at the Salvation Army. Teresa's mother complained of back pain and would frequently quit a job to retire to bed. The back pain was chronic and, medically, no known organic etiology could be found, but she always had the intention of maintaining a job "as soon as her back was better." The mother often would ask Teresa to stay at home when she was in bed. When the mother was not working, she received financial support from AFDC. She moved frequently from one apartment to another and was always without a telephone.

Teresa's father was largely absent from her life; she attempted to develop a relationship with him even though each encounter left her feeling abandoned. He would occasionally contact her but invariably disappointed her by failing to follow through with promises.

Her paternal grandmother, maternal grandmother, and maternal step-grandfather lived in Tennessee. Teresa's mother and the children would travel to the Tennessee farm throughout the year, as often as once a month or more, whenever they felt they could not cope with their lives in Cincinnati. The farm consisted of several dwellings on a homestead, a garden, and some livestock. Teresa's mother also felt that she needed to go to Tennessee to take care of her mother. When one of the grandparents had a heart attack, Teresa's mother packed up her children to move back for a long stay. They were always unclear about how long each visit would be; the stated intention was usually that they would go for the weekend, but they would often stay for a few weeks. On average, they would travel to the farm a dozen times a year. The family viewed the grandparental homeplace as the "real" home for them. Teresa's nuclear family in essence was biresidential, maintaining two equally important residences throughout the entire year.

*Hospital Course.*On the day of Teresa's admission to the adolescent psychiatric inpatient unit, she screamed, cried, and begged her mother not to leave her. The difficulty of this separation was persistent, as she was barely able to tolerate being away from her mother. She felt unsafe when apart from her mother and was afraid something awful would happen to the family. Later in the hospitalization, while at home on a pass, she refused to return to the hospital. She could tolerate being away from her mother for twenty-four hours to avoid hospitalization but had great difficulty managing this anxiety while in the hospital.

Teresa was also depressed, with impaired sleep and appetite, as well as fatigue. Her affect was labile; her behavior was impulsive. The suicidal thoughts that led to taking a drug overdose improved while she was hospitalized, though she intermittently entertained suicidal thoughts. In addition to feeling depressed, she was also explosive. When she broke up with her boyfriend, for example, she found a razor blade and threatened to hurt herself and staff members. She had consistent difficulty following the rules on the unit; she became angry when asked to obey them. Her hospitalization included individual, family, and group sessions to diminish her fears and depression and strengthen the mother's ability to function as a parent. Medication was not used.

By the end of the six-week hospitalization, Teresa's mother felt fortified to help Teresa and Teresa was less anxious and depressed. Some of the symptoms did not resolve, however, and outpatient treatment was suggested to provide further support for the family.

MARY LOU

Mary Lou is also a sixteen-year-old Caucasian adolescent. She had been referred by her school to a psychiatric clinic because of a school phobia. At the first session, she told the psychiatrist that, if forced to return to school, she would kill herself. Because of the suicide threat, she was hospitalized on the university hospital's inpatient adolescent psychiatric service. Mary Lou's truancy from school was sufficient to warrant the school counselor to refer her to juvenile court. She had no prior psychiatric treatment.

*Family History.*At the time of admission, Mary Lou lived with her mother, stepfather, and toddler stepbrother in an urban Appalachian neighborhood. She was born in a West Virginia coal mining town, where her biological father had worked in the mines. Her grandmother took care of Mary Lou while her mother worked. Her mother was divorced when Mary Lou was about six months old and remarried shortly thereafter. After the divorce, Mary Lou's biological father went to live in Kentucky, while Mary Lou, her mother, and stepfather migrated to Cincinnati. The move was precipitated by her stepfather's need to work, as he was unemployed in West Virginia. There was no history of drug use, sexual abuse, or known psychiatric disorder in the family.

Mary Lou was the first person in her family to enter high school; her mother had completed the eighth grade. Mary Lou started her elementary school years in West Virginia where her grandmother expected perfection. If she brought home an *A*, for example, her grandmother would demand to know the exact number grade and would question her if her score was not 100. The grandmother treated her as someone special and Mary Lou felt disappointed about not meeting her grandmother's expectations for perfection.

Mary Lou was truant for ten out of her eleven school years. Throughout this period, she alone would journey back and forth between West Virginia and Cincinnati, reenrolling in school in West Virginia and later leaving to return to Cincinnati, where she would maintain attendance for a short while. At the time of her admission, she was in her junior year, maintaining a straight *A* average, and on the honor roll. Her peer relationships in school appeared normal; she was respected by her friends. She engaged in extracurricular activities, such as participating on the track team and working in the school office. When asked why she felt the need to leave school, she expressed the need to get home for fear something would happen. She felt that "the world was not a safe place, that you simply had to keep a low profile, or something out there would be your downfall." She felt that her strength was within her family and her only sense of safety was within her family. Mary Lou also frequently expressed the need to "get away" and would request of her mother that she be allowed to go to West Virginia. The mother would oblige.

Mary Lou's mother talked about how hard it was for her to leave West Virginia and move to Cincinnati, away from home. The mother had not made any friends and did not work. She sent Mary Lou to do the grocery shopping and family errands. The mother talked about being transplanted and not yet knowing her way around. While Mary Lou was in the hospital, her mother made frequent phone calls stating that she needed Mary Lou at home. Mary Lou was seen as her mother's support; her mother feared danger in the neighborhood and feared telling her own mother that Mary Lou was in the hospital. Mary Lou's mother would look to her to act as the parent to her two-year-old. Mary Lou regarded the toddler as a mother would, watching the child reach developmental milestones.

Hospital Course. On the day of her admission to the hospital, Mary Lou was panicky and very hostile and dictatorial with her mother. She told her mother that she would never speak to her again if she were admitted to the hospital. The mother was crying, the toddler brother was climbing on the furniture, and the mother seemed unable to deal with the situation. When the mother signed the consent forms for treatment, Mary Lou went from being irate to being almost completely withdrawn. She was extremely anxious, she read and reread her Bible, and she remained withdrawn. She was seen as being both rigid and emotionally labile, possibly involving a thought disorder. In the hospital unit, Mary Lou would preach to the other adolescent patients about their use of curse words, their disrespect for one another, and their lack of attention to religion. Overriding all of this was her pleading with all members of the staff to discharge her because she was needed at home. Mary Lou constantly begged for passes from the hospital, especially on the toddler's birthday.

What ultimately altered Mary Lou's behavior was the understanding of Mary Lou's plight by her primary nurse. Mary Lou then lost much of her rigidity. They began to talk about her life in the rural setting, and she began to explain how she felt.

On the ward, Mary Lou initially spent a great deal of time in her room. In addition to the individual, family and group sessions, her treatment included planning time away from home and her mother when on passes from the hospital. Members of her treatment team also worked with her school to develop a plan for her to attend classes until 1:00 p.m. She could tolerate this time away from her mother and continue her education. Following this, she and her mother were able to negotiate how Mary Lou was going to function in the world. Mary Lou set some limits with her mother about her responsibilities in the family, and her mother was able to set some limits with her daughter.

HOMEPLACE TIES

In both cases, the patients and their families made repeated, often extended, visits to their rural places of origin. In Teresa's case, the visits to the Tennessee farm were frequent: once a month, sometimes for several weeks at a time. The visits were always precipitated by a crisis in the family. Teresa's family regarded the rural homestead as a healing place, a place to reconnect with the extended family and with the land. They saw the farm as a place in which to discard, at least temporarily, the tensions and pressures of urban life, including school and employment. There is ambivalence as well: for example, Teresa's mother describes the rural homeplace as a terrible place and comments, "I need to stay here [in Cincinnati]." Mary Lou is under different pressures in West Virginia than in Cincinnati, but she also feels ambivalence toward the rural environment. The ambivalence is not a contradiction but an expression of actual conflicts experienced by the adolescents and their families, especially their mothers.

In fact, the visits to Tennessee and West Virginia caused real conflicts for both families. School truancy was exacerbated. Teresa's mother was unable to work at a job for any length of time even though she was able to acquire numerous positions. The visits also played a positive role in the lives of Teresa's and Mary Lou's families, both psychologically and economically. Teresa's nuclear family moved frequently in Cincinnati, often staying only a few months in one apartment without a phone. The rural homeplace provided temporary residential stability and security, easy communication with the extended family, and a relatively solid economic resource base upon which to draw.

The regularity with which Teresa's family returned to Tennessee was related to scarce resources in the urban environment. They would travel to Tennessee during the latter part of the month, when their monthly check from AFDC had been depleted. The Tennessee farm, while not large or devoted to cash crops, did raise livestock (pigs) and contained a substantial vegetable garden. People could eat well by consuming both preserved foods and fresh vegetables in season.

As a result of the regular visits to Tennessee, however, both Teresa and her mother attempted to live simultaneously in two different worlds, the rural and urban. Teresa's grandmother demanded her daughter (Teresa's mother) to take care of her. Under these conditions, the mother was unable to keep her job in Cincinnati; her reliance upon the welfare system was significant and had a destructive effect upon her self-esteem and the self-esteem of the family. In Tennessee, where both emotional and economic resources were more plentiful, life was seemingly easier. In the long run, however, the more time the family spent in Tennessee, the more difficult it was for them to adapt to urban life. Complicating the picture, however, are the facts that Teresa's mother also left some of her jobs because she regarded her children's problems as more pressing or because she "had a bad back" and required rest.

That Teresa's mother was always unclear as to the length of the visit to the Tennessee homestead is indicative of several complex processes operating in the dynamics of the extended family. These processes include a system of intergenerational reciprocity and one of gender reciprocity (Beaver 1986). Mothers help their daughters when they cannot cope and vice versa. Teresa's grandmother provides food and shelter to her "urban" daughter and her daughter in turn helps her parents when they are ill or when they need other services performed for them, such as helping with harvesting, planting, etc. There is pressure to remain in the rural culture because there is always work to be done. Thus, the time frame is ambiguous for their visits. Teresa's mother may intend to stay only for the weekend, but actually her visits are much longer.

Although Mary Lou has more autonomy than Teresa to determine if and when she visits the rural homeplace, they both experience similar conflicts with respect to their rootedness in the urban environment. In both cases, the rural culture affects them in the city by placing demands on their mothers. The adults realize that they can have their life demands met more easily in the rural setting, either by going to the country themselves, as in the case of Teresa, or by sending their offspring, as in Mary Lou's case. The break with the countryside, at best, is difficult and incomplete. Like their mothers, the patients are both drawn to the rural home. "Home," however, turns out to be problematic, both psychologically and culturally. In Teresa's case, the cultural idiom, home as a safe place, becomes transformed into home as an unsafe, unhappy place; Teresa ran away from her urban home. Mary Lou runs to her grandmother in West Virginia to escape her urban home, but her grandmother's demands weaken her sense of self and impede her adolescent development.

ADOLESCENTS AS CULTURE BROKERS

Both Teresa and Mary Lou mediate between the rural and the urban cultures, but in different ways. They both operate at the interface between two conflicting systems. Several variables can be used to understand the nature of the conflicts. A major one, which directly affects one's ability to cope in an urban environment, is language. Both Mary Lou and Teresa speak a dialect of English that is closer to standard English than that of their mothers. Mary Lou's skills in written English are quite good and Teresa's social skills are strong. Both Teresa and Mary Lou can "pass" as Cincinnatians, as urbanites, without invoking the "hillbilly" stigma evident in their mothers' speech patterns. Both adolescents also have had more experience with urban institutions at a formative stage of their lives. Both know what to expect on palpably dangerous streets; they have no difficulty understanding what merchants say in ordinary encounters in shops and in service institutions, such as the Price Hill Health Clinic. What is perhaps most damaging psychologically both for the mothers and their adolescent daughters is the fact that they are constantly placed in the position of solidifying old ties and creating new ones, only to have them broken or at least disrupted constantly. The pattern of bilocal residence contributes to this discontinuity.

Mary Lou's role as culture broker is more pronounced than that of Teresa; it is also more problematic for her because it is more damaging psychologically. Before leaving West Virginia, Mary Lou's family had adapted to coal mining as a wage labor system, and her mother had a job as a waitress. Thus, for at least a generation, the family had been dependent upon cash for their livelihood. Mary Lou was cared for by her grandmother, who was an appendage to an already nucleated family structure. Mary Lou's family structure contrasts with Teresa's classic rural three-generation extended family (Bryant 1981, 1983). The implications of this contrast cannot be fully delineated here. It should be mentioned, however, that Mary Lou's nuclear family structure rendered her support system quite shallow. For Teresa, and especially for her mother, there were more people upon whom to rely. For Mary Lou, a great deal more is riding upon her success or failure. Mary Lou is the star upon which her family's trajectory of upward mobility depends. Mary Lou's abilities are symbols of achievement in urban culture. She, unlike her mother, has demonstrated that she can cope with city life. She can achieve in school without attending. She is competent to act as a parent or parent-surrogate. She also runs the errands for her household.

Mary Lou's special status in the family, however, creates multiple problems for her. She receives a great deal of attention from both her grandmother and her mother. Her mother's attentions, however, are time demands, and her grandmother's attentions create feelings of inadequacy no matter how hard she works in school. These unrealistic expectations, on the part of her grandmother, create pressures that she finds confusing. She feels complemented by her grandmother's special treatment. She also feels that her grandmother's demands are punitive and require perfection of her. When Mary Lou falls short of the expectations, she is made to feel she is a disappointment. When she got an *A* but not 100%, for example, she felt disappointed, because she knew her grandmother would not be pleased.

Mary Lou's trips to West Virginia do allow her to escape responsibility for her mother's problems. The family was more functional in West Virginia; her mother had a job, and with the grandmother's help, the family could cope with the everyday tasks of providing for the family and caring for Mary Lou. In the urban setting, different problems were created for Mary Lou. She shared the role of mother for her sibling with her own mother just as her mother and grandmother had also shared the parenting role for Mary Lou in West Virginia. In the urban environment, however, their family structure and their residence pattern was different from that in the country. The nuclear family became geographically isolated, with the grandmother remaining in the country. The mother had no one other than Mary Lou to care for the two-year-old. One wonders how the situation would have been different for Mary Lou and for her mother if the grandmother had moved to Cincinnati with them.

Mary Lou's problems can be seen as an extension of her mother's inability to adapt. Her mother places pressure upon Mary Lou to play a major role in running the household and to function as an adult. Mary Lou reacts to the stress in the urban environment by fleeing to West Virginia, where she can be a child, even though there are other pressures for her to deal with there.

Mary Lou's mother had not developed coping skills in the urban environment. She looked to Mary Lou to make decisions for her, much as she had looked to her own mother for support in the rural environment. What was intergenerational reciprocity in the rural setting becomes transformed into Mary Lou's role as a culture broker in the city. Among other things, the role of culture broker places pressure upon Mary Lou to assume, prematurely, the role of primary decision-maker in the family. Adult mothers become dependent upon adolescent daughters, albeit in different ways. It is this dependence that puts the daughters in their positions as mediators, or culture brokers. The system of dependency reverses the role relationships in the rural environment, in which daughters are subordinate to and dependent upon their mothers until the oldest generation ceases to function normally.

CROSS-CULTURAL COMPARISONS AND IMPLICATIONS

The kinds of questions mental health professionals are beginning to ask about other minority groups in the United States need to be addressed for Appalachian Americans as well, particularly those who are experiencing major transitions in their moves from rural to urban environments. In her chapter "The American Indian Child," Carolyn Attneave (1979) points out that when children are presented for diagnosis, therapy, or preventive intervention, professionals must investigate the patients in the context of their families, kin groups, and communities, including place of residence. For urban Appalachians, a rural past that is only one generation deep places many Appalachian people outside of the mainstream culture.

People who came from rural Kentucky, West Virginia, and Tennessee in the most recent wave of migration,came from the poorest areas and had the most difficult adjustments to make in the city (Schwarzweller and Brown 1970). Borman and Mueninghoff (1983) report that among the twenty-four parents interviewed in lower Price Hill, one named thirty relatives living in the neighborhood; only one out of the twenty-four had no relatives living close by; and most of the respondents named seven or more relatives. Most children in lower Price Hill thus grow up in an environment in which they have sustained interaction with kin who live nearby. Unlike most urban Appalachians in Cincinnati, however, the mothers of the two patient cases had no kin residing in their neighborhoods. In this respect, their families are atypical of urban Appalachians, who tend to relocate near close kin who can provide social and economic support, as well as access to jobs (Borman and Mueninghoff 1983).

The fact that the families of the two hospitalized adolescents are isolated and are nuclear families rather than extended families can be seen to be a factor in the pathology. The lack of social, economic, and psychological support systems created instability and pain for the mothers of the adolescents. Mary Lou's mother, for example, asks the hospital staff to help her make basic family decisions; she does not conceptualize her adolescent as a child because she herself is unsettled.

The mothers of the two adolescents were raised by extended family members. When, however, they became parents and expected their children to reproduce the supporting roles, school truancy was the cost. In the city, with a nuclear family, the mother feels there are not enough people around to help her and so feels that the child cannot attend school. At the same time, grandparents in rural areas feel it is their right to expect help from their adult children during times of illness. There is great pressure to conform to these expectations, although to comply with many of these demands makes it difficult to meet the job demands of the urban setting.

Mary Lou's and Teresa's situations are somewhat different with respect to the different economic adaptations of their families in the rural setting. These differences have implications for the treatment process. For example, although it may have been the case that Mary Lou's family resided at some point on a farm on which the extended family was the unit of production, when we encounter Mary Lou, her family is located in a rural coal mining area in which the family structure is essentially nuclear. Teresa's family, by contrast, is an extended, three-generational rural agrarian family. The kinds of entanglements in which Teresa and her mother become involved are very different from those of Mary Lou. When Teresa's mother says she has to go back to Tennessee to take care of her sick mother, we know that she is not indispensible. Other family members could perform the service for the sick woman. Teresa's mother's compulsion to go back is not a need of the social support system, but either (1) a psychological need of the mother, or (2) a form of reciprocity in which the mother is repaying the grandmother for economic support. Given what we know about social structures in rural Tennessee, especially the fact that in many rural Appalachian areas, a person's sense of self is defined not by achievement but by the ascribed status of his or her family, we can see that Teresa's mother may need to go to Tennessee for psychological reasons, to validate her self-concept (Bryant 1981, 1983).

What is deviant or abnormal in one environment may be an expression of normal behavior in another. A mother who seems to refuse to take the responsibility as a parent by placing someone else in the role (in this case an adolescent) is not deviant in the rural culture if no conflicts are created. What makes Mary Lou's mother's behavior deviant in the urban environment is that her demands create serious conflicts for the child in her decision to remain at home or go to school. Serrano and Castillo (1979) note that, for Mexican-Americans, dependency on the extended family represents adaptive behavior. For the Mexican-American adult to remain in frequent contact with his or her mother is expected behavior. Evidence of distance and aloofness, on the other hand, may represent some form of alienation and even psychopathology.

For the families of the two patients just discussed, the move to the city has meant not prosperity and upward mobility but deprivation and downward mobility. From the point of view of human as well as economic resources, life is much better in the country; there is more living space, more food to eat, and more people for emotional support. The pull of the country is a strong force, both psychologically and economically. At the same time, the mainstream, urban-oriented culture bombards people with images of prosperity in the city. Mainstream culture also views the migrants' returns to the homeplace as separation anxiety rather than as attentiveness to real problems (Looff 1971; Looff and Smith 1969). The mainstream culture's conventional wisdom on separation anxiety in this context also implies a negative stereotype of Appalachians; that is, that they are somehow psychologically deficient and cannot cope (McCoy and Watkins 1981). That they cannot cope in the city is often true, but the reasons have to do with a whole complexity of relationships. Perhaps one of the best analyses of this coping problem is Harriette Arnow's novel, *The Dollmaker* (1954), in which the heroine's coping skills are severely hampered by her move to the city. Gertie is a strong, industrious, intelligent woman whose ability to secure and plan her resource base is wiped out from under her by virtue of her total dependency upon her husband's wages in Detroit. Gertie's conflicts are symbolized in her adolescent daughter's reliance upon an imaginary playmate, and the child is ultimately labeled as crazy for managing her mother's tug-of-war in this way (see Borman 1987).

It should be clear that we depart significantly from the position that Appalachians as an ethnic group are unique (Batteau 1983; Precourt 1983; Warner 1985). Rather, we emphasize the rural, minority status of Appalachian migrants and the resultant powerlessness that leads adolescents to psychopathology in mainstream urban American society.

Developing adaptive strategies in situations of rapid culture contact and change is becoming more and more critical for many populations all over the world. The fact that rural Appalachian adolescents experience simultaneously the transitions from country to city and from childhood to adulthood makes them doubly vulnerable but not, from a cross-cultural perspective, unique. In this paper, we have considered economic factors to understand certain aspects of maladaptive behavior and pathology. The study of mental health problems among urban Appalachian adolescents can provide a model for understanding adolescents in other populations experiencing similar changes.

We have shown how two adolescent girls, when placed in positions of culture brokers, develop psychopathology. Because the mothers of these adolescents are themselves unsettled by the rural to urban transition, and because their family structures and resource bases have changed radically in the move, the two adolescents are at risk.

The role of culture-broker, as classically described in the anthropological literature, requires certain skills, as well as certain resources, both economic and psychological. The psychological skills require a person to switch cultures and to act appropriately while maintaining an intact sense of identity in both urban and rural cultures. Thus, what is required is a strongly formed psychological sense of self which must change constantly. It can be argued that these are adult skills; at best it is extremely difficult, if not impossible, for adolescents to accomplish such frequent and rapid changes. The two patients described here have been forced into these roles and their mental health has been severely compromised.

EPILOGUE

"He wanted a job and there was none. He said he was leaving to go live in Cincinnati. Everyone was upset. They said he should stay. I recall my grandmother crying. I asked my mother why. . . ."

She and her husband Tim and their five children had gone back and forth for years, from Harlan County to Dayton, Ohio. They tried living in Chicago too. "We had a terrible time in Chicago, and I think it hurt my children for life. We were away from all our kin. We were afraid of the streets there. And I had to work along with my husband. We came there to make as much money as we could. We hoped that we could save some, and then go back to Kentucky and maybe work some land that belongs to Tim's daddy." [Coles and Coles 1978, p. 79]

Many questions remain for analysis: among them, the issues surrounding the mental health of male adolescents under similar circumstances. Understanding risk factors for adolescents as they experience changes both intrapsychically and culturally is difficult, at best. We have purposely emphasized the cultural changes in order to draw attention to them. That an understanding of adolescence in a cross cultural framework will be aided by this analysis of two Appalachian young women is part of the long term goal of this research.

NOTES

We wish to thank anthropologists Bob Hunt, for pointing out the pattern of bilocal residence, and Kathy Borman, for lending her expertise in Appalachian studies to this study. Terry Sprowl and Judy Sparks, both nurses on the adolescent service, provided us with detailed descriptions of the behaviors of the two patients. Terry Frye and Betsy Woll helped with the typing. Brian Mueller was an invaluable research assistant and was helped by Margie Cantor.

1. A possible exception here is Danna (1980), who notes that certain categories of migrants, including migrants from traditional rural communities, appear to be most vulnerable to psychocultural stress. Women who migrate from communities in which the traditional female role carries severe psychological deprivation appear to be particularly susceptible to depressive states (Dunkas and Nikelly 1972). She notes also that second-generation migrant children are also at high risk as a result of stress brought on by the conflict between traditional childhood socialization practices and the demands of the urban community (Eisenstadt and David 1956).

2. Henry Shapiro's comments on the problem of the identity and distinctiveness of Appalachian culture make it clear that a precise definition of the region is difficult (1978, 1983, p. 133-34).

3. This clinical impression is that of Marcia Slomowitz, M.D., the attending physician on the adolescent service. It remains to be confirmed by epidemiologic data.

REFERENCES

Arnow, H. 1954. *The Dollmaker*. Lexington: University Press of Kentucky [1985].

Attneave, C.I. 1979. The American Indian child. In *Basic handbook of child psychiatry*, vol. 1, ed. J.P. Call, J.D. Noshpitz, R.L. Cohen, and I.N. Berlin. New York: Basic Books.

Batteau, A., ed. 1983. *Appalachia and America: Autonomy and regional dependence*. Lexington: University Press of Kentucky.

Beaver, P.D. 1986. *Rural community in the Appalachian South*. Lexington: University Press of Kentucky.

Borman, K.M. 1987. Urban Appalachian girls and young women: Bowing to no one. In *Class, race and gender in U.S. education*, ed. Lois Weis. Buffalo: SUNY Press.

Borman, K.M., and E. Mueninghoff. 1983. Lower Price Hill children: Family, school and neighborhood. In *Appalachia and America: Autonomy and regional dependence*, ed. A. Batteau. Lexington: The University Press of Kentucky.

Brody, E.B. 1970. *Behavior in new environments: Adaptation of migrant populations*. Beverly Hills, Calif.: Sage Publications.

Bryant, F.C. 1981. *We're all kin: A cultural study of a mountain neighborhood*. Knoxville: University of Tennessee Press.

Bryant, F.C. 1983. Family group organization in a Cumberland mountain neighborhood. In *Appalachia and America*, ed. A. Batteau. Lexington: University Press of Kentucky.

Coles, R. 1971. *Children in crisis*, vol. 2, *Migrants, sharecroppers, mountaineers*. Boston: Little, Brown.

Coles, R., and J.H. Coles. 1978. *Women of crisis: Lives of struggle and hope*. New York: Delacorte Press.

Danna, J.J. 1980. Migration and mental illness: What role do traditional childhood socialization practices play? *Culture, Medicine and Psychiatry* 4:25-42.

Dunkas, N., and G. Nikelly. 1972. The Persephone syndrome: A study in the adaptive process of Greek female immigrants in the USA. *Social Psychiatry* 7:211-16.

Eisenstadt, S., and B. David. 1956. Intergenerational conflict in Israel. *International Social Science Bulletin* 8(1): 54-75.

Looff, D.H. 1971. *Appalachia's children: The challenge of mental health*. Lexington: University Press of Kentucky.

Looff, D.H., and M.N. Smith. 1969. School phobia in the southern Appalachian region: Crucial importance of early treatment. *Southern Medical Journal* 62:329-35.

McCoy, C.B., and J.S. Brown. 1981. Appalachian migration to midwestern cities. In *The invisible minority: Urban Appalachians*, ed. W.W. Philliber and C.B. McCoy. Lexington: University Presss of Kentucky.

McCoy, C.B., and V.M. Watkins. 1981. Stereotypes of Appalachian Migrants. In *The invisible minority: Urban Appalachians*, ed. W.W. Philliber & C.B. McCoy. Lexington: University Press of Kentucky.

Mead, M. 1928. *Coming of age in Samoa*. New York: Quill [1961].

Offer, D., E. Ostrov, and K.I. Howard. 1981. *The Adolescent: A psychological self-portrait*. New York: Basic Books.

Peterson, A.C., and D. Offer. 1979. Adolescent development: Sixteen to nineteen years. In *Basic handbook of child psychiatry*, vol. 1., ed. J.P. Call, J.D. Noshpitz, R.L. Cohen, and I.N. Berlin. New York: Basic Books.

Philliber, W.W., and C.B. McCoy, eds. 1981. *The invisible minority: Urban Appalachians*. Lexington: University Press of Kentucky.

Precourt, W. 1983. The image of Appalachian poverty. In *Appalachia and America: Autonomy and regional dependence*, ed. A. Batteau. Lexington: University Press of Kentucky.

Schwarzweller, H.K., and J.S. Brown. 1970. Social class origins and psychological adjustment of Kentucky mountain migrants: A case study. In *Behavior in new environments: Adaptation of migrant populations*, ed. E.B. Brody. Beverly Hills, Calif.: Sage Publications.

Schwarzweller, H.K., J.S. Brown, and J.J. Mangalam. 1971. *Mountain families in transition*. Pennsylvania Park: Pennsylvania State University Press.

Serrano, A.C., and G.C. Castillo. 1979. The Chicano child and his family. In *Basic handbook of child psychiatry*, ed. J.P. Call, J.D. Noshpitz, R.L. Cohen, and I.N. Berlin. New York: Basic Books.

Shapiro, H.D. 1978. *Appalachia on our mind: The southern mountains and mountaineers in the American consciousness, 1870-1920*. Chapel Hill: University of North Carolina Press.

Warner, M. 1985. *Recovering from schizophrenia*. London: Routledge and Kegan Paul.

Wolf, E.R. 1956. Aspects of groups relations in a complex society: Mexico. *American Anthropologist* 58:1065-78.

PART V

Problems and Promise in Appalachian Mental Health Service Delivery

14

Conscience and Convenience in Eastern Kentucky

JOHN WHITE

At the turn of the century, the Progressive movement began in an attempt to reform society's dealings with the criminal, the delinquent, and the mental patient. According to Rothman (1980), the movement was largely a failure. The major result in mental health was a cosmetic gesture in which the asylum of the nineteenth century became the hospital of the twentieth century. The inclusion of the inmates of asylums under the medical model—with the implication of disease, treatment, and cure—did not change the policies of incarceration and coercive custodial care. However, under the new banner, old policies could be construed as treatment and for the patient's own good. In good conscience, innovative assaults on the inmate, such as lobotomy and electroshock therapy, could be added to other "treatments," such as coercive custodial care, deadening routine, water cures, and strait-jackets. At the end of the Progressive period, in the 1960s, the population in these hospitals was still receiving coercive custodial care; was still being drawn predominantly from the poor, the uneducated, and the unskilled; and was still being characterized as chronic, showing high rates of recidivism. Sixty percent of the population were inmates for longer than five years and 27 percent for longer than 15 years. The population, for the most part, was out of sight—and out of mind—for the general public. Rothman titled his book on the Progressive period *Conscience and Convenience*, because although the movement started out in good conscience with an optimistic, meliorist intent, the net effect was to extend the power of the institution without making basic changes in ways of managing inmates. In mental health, this meant enlarging the discretionary authority of the mental health administrators, easing commitment proceedings, and bolstering the legitimacy of an institution based on custodial care in the name of treatment. There had been a regression to convenience for persons in charge of institutions.

In the 1950s, however, a change in perspective emerged from the studies on effects of long-term institutionalization. This was comparable to the findings of Semmelweis (Szasz 1973, p. xii), the nineteenth-century Hungarian physician who uncovered the cause of puerperal fever, which killed women and infants following childbirth. He showed that the deaths were not due to the weakness of the women but to the poor hygiene of physicians and midwives. In the case of treatment in mental hospitals, long-term institutionalization was discovered to have iatrogenic (physician induced) effects. Institutionalization was found to cause a degenerative process, leaving the inmate worse than when he or she entered. The inmate was found to become resigned, apathetic, and actually dependent on the institution. The routine was found to be so debilitating and require so little from the inmate that he or she loses most of the social and coping skills brought into the hospital. The long-term inmate would remain sensitive to this plight and, when faced with discharge, might exhibit an acute psychotic episode that ensured continued incarceration.

In this context, on February 5, 1963, President Kennedy presented Congress with a program on mental health and mental retardation. The core of the program was to make care for the mentally distressed and retarded available in every community. A related aim was to reduce the large population in the mental hospitals and alleviate the iatrogenic effects. The program was designed to close the gap between the institutions and the community to solve the constant problem of reentry. The gap was to be closed by outpatient clinics, halfway houses, inpatient wards in local general hospitals, follow-up programs, and education programs in the community. The mental hospital was to become a last resort.

Kentucky provided an ideal locale to try the brave goals of the program. Eastern State Hospital in Lexington, founded in 1824, was the first state asylum west of the Appalachians and the second in the United States, preceded only by Virginia's asylum at Williamsburg. In the 1960s, it was overcrowded and understaffed, serving many Kentucky counties notorious for poverty. Federal funds came easily and the Comprehensive Care Program developed there became a model for many other states.

The general plan, designed by the Kentucky Mental Health Planning Commission, specified:

In specific reference to the treatment of mental illness a Comprehensive Community MH-MR Complex should provide at least five essential services:

1. Inpatient care. This unit offers treatment to patients needing 24 hour care.

2. Outpatient care. This unit covers treatment programs for adults, children, and families.

3. Partial hospitalization. This unit offers, at least, day care and treatment for patients able to return home evenings and weekends. Night care may also be provided for patients able to work but in need of further care or without suitable home arrangements.

4. Emergency care. 24 hour emergency services available in one of the three units named above.

5. Consultation and education. These services to community agencies and to professional personnel must be available.

In order to achieve a truly complete comprehensive community mental health center these additional services would be included:

6. Diagnostic service. This service provides diagnostic evaluation, and may include recommendations for appropriate care.

7. Rehabilitation service. This service includes both social and vocational rehabilitation. It offers for those who need them services such as pre-vocational testing, guidance counseling, and sometimes job placement.

8. Pre-care and after-care. This service provides screening of patients prior to hospital admission, and home visiting before and after hospitalization. Follow-up services for homes and halfway houses.

9. Training. This program provides training for all types of health personnel.

10. Research and evaluation. The Regional Board must establish methods for evaluating the effectiveness of its program. It may also carry out research into mental illness or cooperate with other agencies in research. [1966, pp. 56-57]

For all the optimistic, meliorist intent, President Kennedy's program would not have gone anywhere without two less noble facts: first, the cost of "hospitalization" was high and federal grants were readily available for community programs; second, in the 1950s new, mood-altering drugs became available. The drugs of the phenothiazine family were quickly followed by antidepressants, the minor tranquilizers, and lithium salts. The phenothiazines dampen acute psychotic episodes and reduce hallucinations, delusions, and mood swings. The antidepressants reduce depression and the likelihood of suicide. The minor tranquilizers reduce anxiety and physiological arousal. The lithium salts control the extreme mood swings of the manic depressive. In general, they dramatically reduce the behavioral problems exhibited by people with mental problems. This is primarily a cosmetic effect, however, more a convenience to others than a bene-

fit to the patient. Drug therapy tends to mask problems while producing a subdued, more manageable person. The conscience of the
movement was undergirded by the lower cost of outpatient care and
the convenience of an inexpensive chemical straitjacket.

Although the foregoing is important when considering the Comprehensive Care Program, other generally accepted facts about low-
income people and mental health care should be mentioned. Throughout the United States the lower one's socioeconomic status, the more
likely that person is to be committed for a severe mental disorder,
the longer the stay is likely to be, and the greater are the chances of
returning. In rural areas, lower levels of income and education are
combined with higher levels of general ill health and mental disorders,
fewer qualified professionals and difficult access (travel) to facilities.
A less-educated population, in addition, is less likely to seek help
with mild disturbances, so many have their first contact with the
mental health establishment only when severely disturbed.

COMPREHENSIVE CARE IN EASTERN KENTUCKY

Eastern Kentucky has long been considered a dramatic example of a
depressed region. Unemployment, disease, mental retardation, low
educational levels, unstable economy, and marginal agriculture are
continuing problems. Many researchers describe unique subcultural
characteristics based on its history, population, and geography.

Attempting to define the problems faced and the population
served, I surveyed the literature on mental health in the Appalachian
region and spoke with twenty-three mental health professionals at
ten different sites in Eastern Kentucky. Eleven of these professionals
were Eastern Kentucky natives. What follows brings together in a
summary fashion impressions from the interviews and the survey of
available literature. The persons interviewed cannot be held responsible for the summary or the analysis, in as much as I have imposed
my own selective interpretation on the material.

The practitioners surveyed were primarily social workers, clinical
psychologists, and psychiatric nurses with CompCare of Kentucky.
They appeared a competent cadre who performed well in a difficult
situation; but they indicated that staff morale can be a problem, owing
to the extent of their clients' personal and social problems.

The client population comes almost entirely from lower-income
ranges. A client may be in a family where mental retardation, poor
nutrition, chronic disease, mental disturbance, alcoholism, incest, and

spouse abuse are interwoven in a context of chronic unemployment, low education, and geographic isolation. One practitioner said she did not always know where to start. A client may be referred for a psychological evaluation and only incidentally report that she is a victim of incest and frequent beatings. This is not a "walk in" population. Most are referred to a center through the courts, the Bureau of Social Services, a mental hospital, the schools, or a medical clinic. Almost all the clients are subsidized through state or federal funds.

There is a big difference between the perceptions of the CompCare practitioner and those of the clients concerning the nature of services. CompCare practitioners are fully socialized representatives of contemporary culture with a high degree of psychological sophistication. The contemporary "psychological person" has a vast store of words, concepts, and implicit understandings that are signs of this sophistication. Madness and sanity are not seen as dichotomous but as extreme positions on a continuum. Lives are seen as full of inner conflicts (conscious and unconscious), interpersonal conflicts, and conflicts with institutions. The conflicts are conceived of in psychological terms. The contemporary society includes psychiatrists, psychoanalysts, clinical psychologists, psychotherapists, psychiatric social workers, school psychologists, psychiatric nurses, counseling psychologists, educational psychologists, psychometricians, marriage and family therapists, and, a relatively new example, the community psychologists. This sophistication is so pervasive that critics say we are trying to turn ordinary human suffering into a "psychological problem" that can be solved (Gross 1978, p. 6). Blount (1982, p. 77) wryly suggests that trying to live without a sense of original sin makes us need psychiatrists.

However one may feel about this, psychological sophistication is a part of contemporary society and a communication problem occurs when working with the low-income population in Eastern Kentucky because the people lack this sophistication. The client population in the centers holds a dichotomous view of mental problems. One is either "crazy" and gets shipped to Eastern State Hospital, or one is sane. If one is sane, then one does not have mental problems. Typical clinical problems involving anxiety or depression are experienced in a somatic or constitutional framework. "Nerves" is a common complaint: "I got bad nerves," or "Broke my nerves working in the mines." One man reported that he had had his nerves "removed" in an operation.

The typical client not actively psychotic exhibits depression with chronic anxiety. He or she is passive and dependent, with a variety of generalized somatic complaints, such as fatigue; trouble sleeping; heart, lung, and chest pains; gastrointestinal difficulties; and problems with fainting, dizziness, and trembling. For more extensive discussions of the phenomenon of "nerves" see Ludwig and Forrester (1981) and Van Schaik (Chapter 6).

A similar phenomenon is the "Eastern Kentucky syndrome" described by Segal (1973, p. 68). The syndrome includes "bad nerves," moderate depression, various aches and pains, vague complaints about heart and lungs, and spells of feeling "smothered." The client is typically an unemployed man who does not qualify for workman's compensation, social security, or welfare because of the low level of disability. Because of his complaint about "nerves" he ends up getting a psychological evaluation and a prescription for anxiety or depression. It is suggested that being sick or disabled is a way of adjusting to the frustration of unemployment.

A related phenomenon is suggested in Looff's *Appalachia's Children* (1971), where he reports cases of classical conversion hysteria and hysterical personalities that have not been observed since the 1930s outside of rural areas and low-income populations without much psychological sophistication. These cases involve a denial of psychological difficulties on the part of the client in spite of conflicts apparent to others. The conflicts are expressed by the client in a body language often symbolic of the actual problem. There may be impairments such as blindness, deafness, or paralysis associated with things that are not to be seen, heard, or enacted. These physical blockages are differentiated from actual organic impairments by the lack of any actual disease, lesion, or infection and by the failure of the blockage to follow known anatomical or physiological patterns. The client may exhibit a mild indifference to the impairment. In the Freudian framework, the client has converted a psychological conflict into a physical problem that allows avoidance of the real problem. This type of client traditionally is not analytical, is emotionally immature, and tends to use defenses of denial and repression in a global way.

Looff also reports many psychophysiological reactions—such as vomiting, headaches, stomach and digestive difficulties, fainting, ulcers, asthma, and so on—where the cause seems primarily emotional rather than physical. In both the client with a conversion disorder and the client with a psychophysiological reaction, the presenting complaint is physical and any suggestion that the problem is psychological is resisted and may precipitate termination of the contact.

CompCare practitioners spontaneously confirm reports in the literature; what emerges is a picture of psychologically unsophisticated clients exhibiting little insight into personal and interpersonal dynamics. Mental problems are experienced as physical, and medical diagnosis, treatment, and cure are sought. This is reinforced with the ready social acceptance of some kind of physical ailment such as "nerves." Their problems are not "mental," because they are not "crazy."

Several practitioners suggest a familiar psychological pattern: denial of personal and interpersonal difficulties until the pressure builds up and unexpressed feelings burst out in episodes of heavy drinking, violence, and other impulsive behavior. The cause for any antisocial behavior is projected outward in blaming something or someone else.

Eastern Kentucky CompCare practitioners also report that most clients take a passive-dependent approach to the contact. The staff members, regardless of professional background, are often referred to as "Doctor" by the client, and the client appears to want a diagnosis and "treatment" involving "medicine" that will lead to a "cure." The notion of actively struggling with one's problems, required in most psychotherapy, is not present and must be carefully developed if it occurs at all.

The picture presented above is not without stigma in the eyes of middle-class mainstream Americans. A low-income uneducated person who has problems he or she won't admit, who is impulsive and acts up, who won't come in for treatment unless coerced, who doesn't try to help the psychotherapist, and who only wants medicine for "nerves" is not an attractive client.

A survey of rural attitudes toward mental health in North Carolina (Lee, Gianturco, and Eisdorfer 1974) confirms this view of the population. The authors complain that the clients resist coming in for help, and report that the population does not usually know the centers exist. When the center's existence is known, people do not understand the services, and when they do understand, they avoid the centers until the problem is acute.

By shifting to the clients' point of view, we may see the wisdom in avoiding CompCare Centers. They are places where the poor and powerless are sent for labeling. When labeled, clients are then shipped to Eastern State Hospital or "treated" locally, often against their will. Even entering the center makes one suspect. In one community, the center is in a trailer across the street from the county courthouse. Anyone going in passes through the busy communication center of the town.

The CompCare centers, in fact, are an extension of the local political establishment and evoke suspicion. In the center, decisions are made about commitments, voluntary and involuntary. It is where one is sent for "treatment," if one comes up before the judge for alcohol and drug abuse or for spouse and child abuse—if one doesn't want to go to jail. It is where other branches of government send assorted low-income, problem cases. It is where ex-mental patients and people with "nerves" go. Why go near the place at all? If one is sent there, why not be passive, play along, and keep a low profile? And why not admit to some vague physical problems, so the relationship can be managed in a mutually beneficial way? The low-income client probably knows the system and has been trained by experience. The client also might have good reason for getting drunk, taking drugs, and "acting up." What is seen as a lack of psychological sophistication by middle-class Americans may be, in some cases, a client's astute grasp of the reality of powerlessness. This view of reality might reflect the subtle wisdom imputed to peasant and slave societies, where one avoids making oneself available for the ministrations of the local establishment.

One should not become too romantic about the poor, for expressions of psychological problems may be suppressed for other reasons. Discussions of a psychological nature may be avoided in the center so that the client may escape being mistaken for one who has psychological problems. Someone with close family ties and a strong church affiliation does not take family problems out of the family or church without a sense of disloyalty. Another factor may be the stoicism attributed in the literature and by practitioners to inhabitants of the region. Discussion of problems is an admission of weakness and a burden to the hearer. Finally, an unemployed person with little education, from an isolated region and suffering from poor nutrition may simply not be as cognitively complex and sophisticated as middle-class Americans.

One can say, with considerable assurance, that there is a difference between the perspective of the typical middle-class American and the typical client in a CompCare Center. This presents a problem in itself, but there is potential for even greater difficulty when such a difference in attitude is linked with a difference in social power and influence. Jacquelyn Murray suggests a grim scenario as a result of her research:

While working at a state hospital where Appalachians were being hospitalized, it seemed to this investigator that they were being hospitalized for behaviors described in the literature as normative to their culture. Often the behaviors precipitating admission included impulsive behaviors such as fighting, drinking, domestic quarrels or child abuse. The diagnostic symptoms most frequently cited were withdrawal, flattened affect, impoverished speech patterns, paranoia, hostility, poor impulse control and apathy. These behaviors bear a striking resemblance to those used to describe normative Appalachian temperament: stoic and non-communicative, suspicious and distrustful of outsiders, fatalistic and pessimistic, hostile toward outsiders and having an action orientation. [1979, pp. 41-42]

Murray's observations led her to compare how Appalachians and non-Appalachians view people with problems. Murray developed a series of behavioral vignettes describing problematic behavior. The vignettes were based on actual case histories of Appalachian clients hospitalized and diagnosed as mentally ill in Chicago. These vignettes were used as a basis for a structured interview with a representative sample of Appalachians, mental health practitioners, and a lay group of non-Appalachians, all from the Chicago area. Although there was no significant difference between lay non-Appalachians and mental health professionals in their interpretations of the vignettes, these groups differed significantly from the Appalachians. The first two groups readily labeled the behavior as mental illness. The Appalachians did not and used totally different categories for the behavior. They might describe the person in the vignette as lazy, mean, immoral, or criminal, but not as crazy. They also made quite different recommendations for treatment.

CONVENIENCE CLOSES IN

As suggested earlier, the dramatic reduction in the inmate population during the 1960s owed as much to the new psychotropic drugs as to community mental health centers. Now, many inmates could be maintained via drug therapy in their homes and communities.

Until the 1950s psychiatry had been struggling to justify its existence within the medical profession with crude treatment such as electroshock therapy, insulin shock therapy, lobotomy, and a few sedatives. The software—such as psychoanalysis, psychotherapy, group therapy, and the various supplements—did not help psychiatry and its image, because these treatments could be administered by psychologists, social workers, and nurses. With the discovery, in rapid sequence, of an array of powerful psychotropic drugs in the 1950s, psychiatry came into its own. It now had medications to treat mental illness, and these medications apparently produced dramatic cures. Now, psychiatry would no longer have to be the weak sister of physical medicine, and it would not have to compete with nonmedical personnel, because prescriptions are written only by physicians. Today, Sterling (1979) reports, "psychotropic drugs have become virtually the universal and sole treatment for mental patients" (p. 14).

The institutional use of the major tranquilizers or antipsychotic drugs (phenothiazines like Thorazine and Stelazine, and butyrophenones like Haldol and Prolixin) made possible the end of the straitjacket, padded cells, and other forms of physical restraint. The acutely psychotic inmate could be "snowed." Antidepressants (tricyclics like Elavil and Vivactil, and monoamine oxidase inhibitors like Nardil and Parnate) helped reduce the surveillance necessary for depressed inmates. The minor tranquilizers (benzodiazepines like Valium and Librium) made the anxious, fearful, phobic inmate less disruptive and distressing. Lithium salts made it possible to buffer the disruptive highs and lows of the manic depressive. These drugs were a tremendous boon and, with or without mental health centers, many persons previously unacceptable to their families and community could be sent home. Conscience was satisfied inasmuch as the best of modern scientific medicine was being applied, and patients were being treated at home. And all that was required was a prescription and someone to administer medicine.

Today we know that these medicines are toxic, and contemporary Semmelweises are awakening those who will listen. With the major tranquilizers, the first side effects include a dry mouth, blurred vision, and the inability to ejaculate. There is often trembling of the limbs and rigidity of muscle groups leading to an inability to move (akinesia). Fidgeting, pacing, twitching, and a general inability to get comfortable (akathisia) are also frequent. There are even occasional attacks of intense anxiety and terror, usually ascribed to the client's "illness." These side effects are managed by prescribing more drugs. Long-term dosages produce tardive dyskinesia, characterized by rhythmic and involuntary movements of the tongue, face, mouth, and jaw. The arms and legs may also be affected. This iatrogenic disorder is irreversible, a sign of permanent brain damage (Goldstein, Baker, and Jamison 1980, p. 153). Treatment is to prescribe more drugs. The patient is now unmistakably stigmatized, and the layman thinks the grotesque movements are mental illness.

Mark Vonnegut gives this first-person account of drug therapy:

Taking Thorazine was part of doing things right. I hated Thorazine but tried not to talk about hating it. . . . But Thorazine has a lot of unpleasant side effects. It makes you dizzy and faint when you stand up too quickly. If you go out in the sun your skin gets red and hurts like hell. It makes muscles rigid and twitchy. The side effects were bad enough, but I liked what the drug was supposed to do even less. It's supposed to keep you calm, dull, uninterested, and uninteresting. . . . What I think it does is just fog up your mind so badly you don't notice the hallucination or much else. . . . On Thorazine everything's a bore. Not a bore exactly. Boredom implies impatience. . . . When I did manage to get excited about some things, impatient with some things, interested in some things, it still didn't have the old zing to it. [1976, pp. 252-53]

The initial claim for chemical therapy was that these drugs would make a person more amenable to psychotherapy. We now know that, although more acute symptoms like hallucinations can be reduced, the associated blunting of consciousness, of motivation, and of problem-solving ability does not aid the psychotherapeutic process.

One CompCare practitioner who runs a day-care center for clients on the major tranquilizers said that none of the clients like the medication, but they know they will "get into trouble" if they don't take them. Another practitioner reported that the parents of a thirty-year-old client requested that their daughter's medicine be increased, because she was getting out of her chair three and four times a day and drinking too much iced tea. For obvious reasons the involuntary use of drugs has now been successfully challenged in the courts (Sterling 1979), but there are many ways to coerce. One threat for the client stubborn about medication is that of sending him or her back to the hospital. Or a client uncooperative about the oral doses is told that Prolixin will be substituted. Prolixin is given in the form of a timed-release injection that lasts for a period of two weeks. Most clients know Prolixin has pronounced side effects, among them an occasional muscle spasm that causes the tongue to protrude six to eight inches. A practitioner reported that one of her day-care clients suddenly disappeared, and when located was hiding in the broom closet with her hand clamped over her mouth. Concerned about what the client might have in her mouth, the practitioner pulled away the client's hand and her tongue jutted out at full extension. The client seemed aware it would be difficult to improve her interpersonal relations or her self esteem while stigmatized in this fashion.

The abuse of medication is often in the hands of the caretaker. If caretakers are overworked or uninterested, the strain between what is helpful to the client and what is convenient is accentuated. Some families feel burdened by the client. The centers suffer major reductions in staff. The initial federal grants have run out and the state governments have not taken up the slack.

In the case of less severely disturbed clients, the dialectic between conscience and convenience is less strained. These clients are likely to be taking the most widely prescribed psychotropic drug, a minor tranquilizer (usually Valium or Librium). It is also the most widely abused prescription drug in the country today (Hughs and Brevin 1979), and Garr (1979) reports that enough Valium is produced to provide each person in the United States with 100 pills a year. In a recent movie, *Starting Over*, a comedy scene was staged in Bloomingdale's in New York City. In a minor emergency one character asks the onlookers, "Does anybody have a Valium?" and each person offers one.

Although minor tranquilizers are widely used and abused throughout the United States, the typical user is not under any illusion about having a disease Valium will cure. In Eastern Kentucky, the typical low-income client with mental problems experiences the problem as "nerves," and "nerve medicine" does give a form of relief.

There is a shortage of physicians as well as mental health practitioners in Eastern Kentucky, and when a client appears with vague, generalized, somatic complaints that sound psychological to the physician, a prescription takes about 30 seconds to write, whereas medical pursuit of the complaints could take considerably longer and end in frustration. The combination of a harried physician and a stressed client with "nerves" couldn't be handled with more finesse than with "nerve" pills. How can one argue with a satisfied patient and relieved doctor, especially when the transaction takes place within the comfortable paradigm of disease, treatment, and cure? The transaction is further legitimized by government funding, which pays the bill. Conscience and convenience are collapsed into a pill—and tranquil people don't cause problems.

It would be easy to say that a conspiracy was afoot, that "firewater" is pushed in what Peter Schrag once called our "vast paleface reservation," in order to keep the natives quiet and happy. It is more likely something as banal, if more threatening, as available technology, narrow professionalism, and a need to solve problems efficiently.

The long-standing deep-seated fear of the deviant has not lessened.

The response is just more sanitary and duplicitous. When the madmen were locked up in asylums, we were safe. With a provoked conscience, the asylum was renamed hospital and treatment continued in the same fashion. With a conscience pricked once again, convenient chemicals called medicine were used to make the deviant seem more like others and thus less threatening. In low-income, culturally different regions, two birds could be killed with one stone: treating the deviant and the poor with the best medicine. And their different perspective on mental problems makes them willing confederates.

Community mental health centers face a difficult situation: a population not prepared to accept the center's nonmedical service, a reduced staff, and a chemical folie á deux between the local physician and the client that undercuts the center's efforts with less disturbed clients. It also appears that, although the centers were developed as a substitute for incarceration, via outpatient drug therapy, they are often an efficient supplement to incarceration and allow even more persons to be kept under control. When conscience and convenience clash, convenience usually wins, and people move closer to the hospital society Goethe predicted (cited in Rieff 1966, p. 24).

REFERENCES

Blount, R. 1982. *Crackers*. New York: Knopf.

Garr, D. 1979. Getting drugs: By hook or by crook. *Family Health* (November):29.

Goldstein, M.J., B.L. Baker, and K.R. Jamison. 1980. *Abnormal psychology*. Boston: Little, Brown.

Gross, M.L. 1978. *The psychological society*. New York: Random House.

Hughs, R., and R. Brevin. 1979. Daze of our lives. *Family Health* (November):28-31.

Kentucky Mental Health Planning Commission. 1966. *Pattern for change*. Frankfort: Author.

Lee, S.H., D.T. Gianturco, and C. Eisdorfer. 1974. Community mental health center accessibility. *Archives of General Psychiatry* 31(September):335-39.

Looff, D.H. 1971. *Appalachia's children*. Lexington: University Press of Kentucky.

Ludwig, A.M., and R.L. Forrester. 1981. The condition of "nerves." *Journal of the Kentucky Medical Association* 79(6):333-36.

Murray, J.H. 1979. *Perceptions of problematic behavior by Appalachians, mental health professionals and lay non-Appalachians*. Ann Arbor, Mich.: University Microfilms.

Rieff, P. 1966. *The triumph of the therapeutic: Uses of faith after Freud*. New York: Harper & Row.

Rothman, D.J. 1980. *Conscience and convenience: The asylum and its alternatives in progressive America*. Boston: Little, Brown.

Segal, J., ed. 1973. *The mental health of rural America*. DHEW Publication No. (HSM) 73-9035. Washington, D.C.: U.S. Government Printing Office.

Sterling, P. 1979. Psychiatry's drug addiction. *The New Republic* 181(December 8):14-18.

Szasz, T.S. 1973. *The age of madness*. Garden City, N.Y.: Anchor Books.

Vonnegut, M. 1973. *The Eden express*. New York: Bantam Books.

15

Mental Health Professionals in Appalachia

MELANIE L. SOVINE

This essay addresses the role of health care professionals in Appalachia, focusing on the delivery of mental health care by psychiatric social workers in Appalachian community mental health clinics. Of particular concern is the relevance of Appalachian studies and clinical anthropology to the practical knowledge utilized by primary therapists in the patient-practitioner encounters that make up a large part of the therapists' clinical day. My purpose is to illustrate the need for a body of literature applicable to health care delivery in Appalachia. Addressing this need involves a refocused perspective on regional professionals, understanding them as individuals whose appropriate education about Appalachia requires renewed efforts. In support of these renewed efforts, let us first consider the predominant perspectives on professionals in Appalachia.

THE PROFESSIONAL CLASSES IN APPALACHIA

Southern Appalachia is a colonial possession of Eastern based industry. Like all exploited colonial areas, the "mother country" may make generous gestures now and then, send missionaries with up-lift programs, "superior" religion, build churches and sometimes schools. They'll do about everything—except get off the backs of the people, and the exploitive domination. That the people themselves must eventually see to. The latest "missionary" move is the "War on Poverty." It was never intended to end poverty. That would require a total reconstruction of the system of ownership, production and distribution of wealth. From their affluent middle class background so many do-gooders who come into the mountains seldom grasp the fact that the poor are poor because of the nature of the system of ownership, production and distribution. When the poor fail to accept their middle class notions they may end up frustrated failures. Some put their frustrations into a book. [West 1972, p. 212]

In Appalachian studies, considerable attention is given to professionals, who, as a social class, are criticized as proponents and implementors of humanistically detrimental, if not destructive, sociocultural changes in the region. The motives and objectives of the professional classes, whether undergirded by benevolence or by the profit motive, are viewed with skepticism, a skepticism related to ethnographically and historically inaccurate stereotypes held by professionals about Appalachian people. These inaccuracies were not only related to professional motivations but problematically became the ideological bases upon which programmatic developments were designed for far-reaching sociocultural changes in Appalachia. These changes, a so-called modernization of the mountain native, who is believed to be maladaptively "traditional," primarily were directed at the Appalachian poor. By the 1960s, the Appalachian-based social programs were among the worst of the War on Poverty, wherein the deficiencies of the people to be benefited by the programs were all too readily agreed upon and publically acknowledged and the realities of the economic structures that actually resulted in the region's poverty and other human miseries were all too carefully unacknowledged and underdisclosed.

A more authentic view of the social and economic history of Appalachia focused attention on the professional classes as the handmaidens of a controlling and capitalizing industrialization of Appalachia (see Lewis, Johnson, and Askins 1978). The corresponding change in attitude toward professionals was a near reversal. At one time, professionals who lived and worked among an "isolated" Appalachian people were revered as interpreters of an exotic experience hardly containable by most Americans. These men and women functioned as primary sources for descriptions of Appalachian history and culture, with a role as the "outside interpreter" familiar to hundreds of lay social workers, early ethnographers, missionaries, and developers who immersed themselves worldwide in cultures otherwise inaccessible to mainstream Americans (Klotter 1980; Prucha 1970; Sovine 1986). When the authenticity of these interpretations was severely challenged and their motivations questioned, regional professionals came to be viewed as a malevolent group who insensitively and selfishly acquiesced to changes nearly destroying the cultural underpinnings of the ethnically and socially diverse Appalachian population, perpetuating through their many publications the degrading images of Appalachians so familiar to other Americans.

Certainly, the intervention by health care professionals into Appalachian health care is a telling episode in the continually emergent story of planned social and cultural change in the region, and the portrayals of Appalachian people written by those with medical and psychological perspectives are among the most degrading and pejorative in print (see, for example, Ball 1968; Finney 1970; Goshen 1970).

Once, during interim employment with a regional hospital corporation, I met with a local hospital administrator, a middle-aged native of Eastern Kentucky who had worked in the region all his life. He handed me an envelope, the contents of which, in some way, he found laughable. Inside was a soiled and badly folded piece of elementary school notebook paper with large and unevenly scrawled words of sincerity and gratitude for care received during a recent hospitalization. It was signed "Charlie." Charlie requested the administrator to extend his gratitude to all caretakers involved in his recent admission. Charlie was a local man, chronically and ambulatorily mentally ill, sometimes delusional, though always lucid in matters of social courtesy. He experienced multiple physical complications associated with his mental illness and with the essentially outdoor life-style he had designed for himself. Maintaining a reasonable amount of personal choice, Charlie lived in his own poorly constructed dwelling. He was often dirty and dishevelled and carried a suitcase, which he said contained telephones that rang directly to the White House. Though in the depths of mental illness and poverty, Charlie was nevertheless a gracious and unassuming man. As social class ironies often go, the administrator, with all the neat and clean accoutrements of middle management, was not. I, therefore, can say that I have known and worked with health care professionals who clearly embody the worst of professional images in Appalachia.

It is too simple, however, to assume that all professionals may be classed collectively as exploitive agents of social and cultural change. Although the systems of inequality and patterns of economic development responsible for the poor quality of life experienced by many Appalachians are wretched, not all professionals working within these systems are to be despised or dismissed as intolerable enactors of injustice. Further, professionals do not neatly fall into a single descriptive category, such as the "outside exploiter" or the "outside interpreter" of Appalachian people (Eller 1983; Thompson and Wylie 1983-1984). In working anew with professionals in Appalachia, we must no longer categorically associate them with detrimental sociocultural change or characterize them categorically as nonlocal authors of a pejorative literature or of social programs based upon such literature. Let us consider further the degree to which Appalachian scholarship may influence health care professionals.

Two primary sources fundamentally shape one's knowledge and feelings about Appalachia: the media and the Appalachian studies literature. Much of this literature today is produced by scholars and activists associated with the Appalachian Studies Conference. The Appalachian Studies Conference has pledged to produce a more authentic appraisal of Appalachian social problems, seeking to encourage social and cultural changes designed to benefit the regions' inhabitants rather than reinforce dependency and social inequality (Fisher, Williamson, and Lewis 1977; McGowan 1982). The conference attempts to integrate individuals working in applied settings with those engaged in regional scholarship. Though the goals are worthy and the efforts sincere, the conference has not been particularly successful in involving nonacademic professionals in the activities of the conference. Regional organizations with less of an academic focus though with similar goals—for example the Commission on Religion in Appalachia (see Couto 1984)—are also available for professional participation, though the laudable efforts of these organizations are largely directed toward grass-roots community organizing around social and economic issues. Very often and understandably, these organizations are at legal and political odds with professional leaders, administrators, and officials in an attempt to resolve social and economic injustices. These organizations have an impressive history of addressing issues related to health care, but this has been directed at the level of health systems development rather than at the level of daily interactive encounters, where most health care professionals are absorbed by the immediacy and density of clinical demands. Health care professionals are likely to have neither the time nor the motivation to attend conferences or participate in organizations not immediately relevant to clinical care.

Although critical thinkers in Appalachian studies have been quick to expose regional stereotypes, to challenge professional motivations, and to reinterpret the Appalachian experience along more authentic economic and social dimensions, the scholarly focus and published literature are also broadly systemic, addressing regional sociopolitical and economic questions that are nationally encompassing. This material is not easily nor always successfully applicable in a work setting like the clinic (Plaut 1983). Moreover, although the worst of the publications once most frequently used by professionals in Appalachia have been severely and effectively criticized (see Fisher 1976; Lewis

1970; Lewis, Koback, and Johnson 1973), the specifics of these criticisms are little known except to Appalachian scholars and a select group of politically sensitive regional activists.

Many health care professionals, particularly those for whom the behavioral sciences were integral components in their training, work in the region having read only the earlier, inaccurate studies of Appalachian communities, social problems, and culture, and having been exposed to the mass media productions on Appalachian poverty. Though it is often assumed otherwise, many of these professionals, both local and nonlocal, are self-educated, particularly about Appalachia. Given their influence on social life in the region, these professionals cannot be dismissed nor disregarded as an important readership for the more recent, critical Appalachian studies literature.

The question is how to more evenly inform professionals with Appalachian studies materials and, in turn, produce materials immediately relevant and easily applicable to the everyday work setting. This requires a change of presentation, for regional scholars and activists have engaged mostly in the production of political commentary and sociocultural analyses of the Appalachian experience; pragmatic and specific literature of use to professionals is sparse. Further, there is a tendency to engage in an "academic scolding" of those who fail to adopt points of view believed to be most appropriate when working in Appalachia. Unfortunately, this scolding is not accompanied by an attempt to intervene instructively in the professional work setting. Such intervention requires the identification of everyday problems, in turn necessitating a problem-oriented research in addition to the broader interpretive and systemic research questions characteristic of Appalachian studies.

CLINICAL ANTHROPOLOGY AND THE MENTAL HEALTH CLINIC

Clinical anthropology is a perspective that helps health practitioners to achieve a more accurate understanding of the patient through a greater appreciation of his or her cultural background (Chrisman and Maretzki 1982; Eisenburg and Kleinman 1980; Helman 1984; Kleinman 1980). The practitioner accordingly includes "clinically relevant ethnographic data" (Chrisman and Maretzki 1982) in his or her package of practical knowledge, thereby using a pragmatic concept of "culture" (Rubinstein 1986) within the clinical setting. The concept is a pragmatic one in the sense that sociocultural dynamics are allowed

for and recognized in the patient-practitioner encounter and are utilized as pertinent considerations in the assessment of symptoms and
the treatment of illness. These encounters are thereby transformed
into settings for negotiation between patient and practitioner, avoiding an encounter wherein the practitioner imposes a biomedical or
disease-oriented interpretation upon the patient's more socioculturally encompassing experience of illness (see Kleinman 1980; Kleinman, Eisenberg, and Good 1978; Lewis 1980). Mental health patients,
for example, bring problems to the clinic relating to the whole of their
daily experiences. The training received by practitioners in conventional health sciences education encourages them to screen out of
clinical decisions the details giving shape to the sociocultural context
in which the experience of mental illness is situated. The lived-in
quality of mental illness is stripped away, leaving the bare and sterile
biomedical and psychiatric facts. The treatment associated with this
reductionism too often contributes to the patient's mental illness. An
ability to acknowledge, legitimize, and effectively address the totality
of a patient's mental illness experience has significant impact upon
the quality of the patient-practitioner encounter and therefore upon
the therapeutic efficacy of mental health care.

The introduction of the concept of culture into clinical practice as
a means for restoring therapeutic efficacy is occurring in two ways.
One is through curricular innovations in health science institutions
that support an attempt to produce practitioners with both sociocultural and biomedical expertise. A second, lesser known way is
through the placement of cultural anthropologists in clinically applied
roles. Cultural anthropologists bring to the clinic a theoretical and
applied sophistication about the concept of culture as well as an ethnographic expertise appropriate for practice in the selected locale. In
the clinic, the anthropologist assumes a consultant or practitioner role
alongside other health care providers, working cooperatively with the
patient in making health care decisions that are equally socioculturally
and biomedically sophisticated. Particularly important is the integrity
given to the patient's view of his or her illness, thereby integrating
him or her into the patient-practitioner encounter as a full partner
rather than a passive receiver of a medical opinion. Within this encounter, all participants present and negotiate with a specialized
knowledge from which an agreed-upon clinical reality of the patient's
illness is discerned.

When awarded a fellowship to support community service in Appalachia, I was interested in the relationship of religion and mental

health as experienced within the Appalachian cultural context. With the fellowship, I planned to accomplish two objectives: first, I planned to work in a consulting role with clinic practitioners, providing expertise on religion in Appalachia, as well as general medical anthropological expertise. Second, I planned to conduct research on the experience of mental illness in Appalachia, focusing on psychiatric cases in which religion played a significant role. These plans worked well with mental health administrators when negotiating entry as a nonmedical practitioner into the health care delivery system. But, at the local clinic, where practitioner needs were at a crisis level, I unexpectedly and quickly was incorporated into a role as primary therapist, accepting a limited case load of carefully and sensitively referred patients from the other therapists. Through this applied role, I gained an appreciation for the activities of the clinic at the most basic level: the daily patient-practitioner encounter. Through the referral process, the therapists' underlying motivation of caring became clear, as did the inherently conflictual reality of their role within this clinic system, a reality thwarting caring in their patient relationships.

THE CONFLICTUAL ROLE OF THE THERAPIST

The local clinic, in a rural, heavily industrialized, Eastern Kentucky county, had approximately six hundred open cases, the majority of which were individual therapy clients. These cases were divided among five therapists, three full-time, one part-time in therapy and part-time in clinic management, and one part-time employee (one day a week). Intermittently, an undergraduate student would accept a limited number of cases for a two- or three-month practicum. Handling so many clients with essentially a skeleton staff was expected of the local clinic by the administration of the greater Community Mental Health System (CMHS), whose concern was with the survival and maintenance of the mental health care delivery system, even at the cost of effective therapy. Such survival depended upon the availability of federal and state funds, which both originated the rural community mental health programs and supported their continuance (see also Yahraes 1971). In order to ensure its survival, the local clinic was expected to take maximum advantage of federal and state monies, utilizing all local staff. The burden of this maximization lay most heavily on the primary therapists, whose job description had little to do with specific treatment modalities but much to do with processing as many clients as possible through the clinic. This was a cyclical exercise, both statistically establishing mental health care needs in the service area and documenting the delivery of service by CMHS to meet these needs. The needs-service statistical portrait was then used to justify the continuance of the mental health care delivery system. Extensive paperwork, all of it subject to audit, was required for reimbursements on federal and state aid patients. These reimbursements, together with United Mine Workers' Association and Southern Labor Union health payments, were the second most important source of CMHS operational funds. Accurate chart work was directly tied to these operating funds, and primary therapists were directly tied to accurate chart work. Therapists, on the one hand, found themselves torn between the needs of system maintenance while functioning as mental health practitioners motivated by a sincere desire to fulfill the needs of those experiencing mental illness. The inherent conflict in this role was exacerbated by the realities of too many clients, too few therapists, and simply not enough time to be both efficiently bureaucratic and effectively therapeutic, to be both keepers of the system and caretakers of the mentally ill.

The clinic is in an industrialized rural county, where few jobs were available other than those associated with the economy of mining, with its characteristically unstable, dramatic boom and bust cycles. Both the therapists and their clients always feared for their jobs. CMHS employees were told upon hiring, and repeatedly each year, that their jobs could not be assured for more than one year. There are few jobs for college graduates in the area, and these are always filled. Loss of their jobs by local therapists therefore meant dramatic changes in their lives, including potential relocation from their native homes. Nonlocal therapists were no less anxious about these uncertainties, for most had "made a home" in the area, and job loss would also entail significant social and emotional losses.

Though often angry and frustrated in their positions (many of the therapists genuinely cared about their practitioner role and felt this role impeded by the political and economic nature of the delivery system) the therapists nevertheless participated in the administrative agenda. The effects of the administrative agenda were many, though most striking was the degree to which it affected the quality and content of the patient-practitioner encounters. In essence, the primary therapists were the health care delivery system (Yahraes 1973) and much of the nature and tone of the health care obtained within the local clinic was set by these therapists. A failure to maintain a sense of therapeutic efficacy was one of the most serious errors in the actual implementation of this rural mental health care system.

Overworked and seriously understaffed, constantly threatened by the loss of their jobs, the therapists had all but quit trying with many of the patients, though continuing to "follow them"—that is, to process patients through the clinic system. Most serious for the quality and goals of psychotherapy, the negotiations and conversations between the patient and practitioner were all but shut down. For all patients, polymedication was a severe problem. It represented an attempt to meet persistent somatic and emotional complaints, an attempt often counteractive to the efficacy of therapy sessions. Therapists sometimes felt the sessions were useful to the patient only as a means by which multiple medications could be easily obtained and continued. The therapy sessions assumed a redundancy, and the "revolving door" image seemed to characterize the patients' and the practitioners' clinical experience.

Regardless of the problems associated with the rural mental health care programs, there are people in Appalachia, as elsewhere, who genuinely are in need of an intermediate and sustaining mental health care as an alternative to inappropriate incarceration or commitment to a state institution. In eastern Kentucky today, mental health care delivery systems such as CMHS are the only available options. Fortunately for mental health patients, practitioners associated with these rural mental health care programs are genuinely concerned with providing care. Their ability, indeed their freedom, to provide this care is constrained by the design of the delivery system itself, and ultimately a radical restructuring of these services is the only desirable option. Until the far-reaching economic and political changes needed to reconstruct these programs can be effected, the currently operative systems, at the daily service level, need to be reworked and improved.

THE USE OF CULTURE IN AN APPALACHIAN CLINIC

And now this illness again which has always affected me so strangely. I'm sure it is underestimated. Just as the importance of other illnesses is exaggerated. This illness doesn't have any particular characteristics; it takes on the characteristics of the people it attacks. [Rilke, 1985, p. 62]

Differing from many clinical settings, a concept of culture was already operative at the Appalachian Community Mental Health Clinic (ACMHC). Local and nonlocal clinic practitioners and support staff members frequently talked about the Appalachian culture, repeating, as an explanation for patient behavior, "It's their culture; people are different down here." This statement communicated two separate though related themes, one having to do with culture and the other with observed or felt differences between the therapists and their Appalachian clients. The concept of culture and its application in the clinic was most often invoked in situations of frustration with clients. For example, though noncompliance is a general problem in health care and not singularly related to geographical locale, the failure of patients to keep regularly scheduled appointments at ACMHC was frequently discussed as an Appalachian trait, something cultural and common, a behavioral trait one could not and should not expect to change. Overattendant patient behavior was also labeled *Appalachian*. These patients, most presenting with vague and chronic complaints such as "bad nerves," were said to display a culturally accepted behavior of visiting multiple physicians, sometimes all in one day, as a sort of social event rather than as a prescribed biomedical or recommended psychotherapeutic event. References to culture, therefore, occurred in discussions about the patients' use of the clinic, and an Appalachian gloss was given to the patterns patient behavior assumed in the course of passing through the clinic. At the same time, references to culture were used in justifying the actions therapists took or the choices made in the routine management of patients. Unable to meet all the patient care demands, the therapists rarely monitored closely the clinic attendance of patients who refused or were unable to consistently maintain a tightly defined clinical care process. Little effort was expended on modifying patient behavior, insisting they attend the clinic according to the steps outlined in the clinic procedures manual. Such an inflexibility, indeed, would have been unreasonable and unrealistic for most of these rural patients and for the understaffed therapists.

When questioned closely about their idea of an Appalachian culture, both native and nonnative therapists made general descriptive comments, all of which they shuffled around a vaguely defined, though clearly felt, sense of difference. Although therapists thought of themselves as working with a cultural group—"Appalachians"—an additional reality about their practice contributed to this sense of difference. These therapists were health care providers to the poor and lower working class. During this research period, the misunderstandings associated with social class differences were escalating to the level of antagonism in the face of general economic decline and on-coming "hard times" and in relation to the community reputation of the clinic as a health care facility for "people who just won't work" and who were using psychiatric disabilities to obtain welfare payments. Therapists were accused of providing free health care to a "no good" group of people.

Both patients and practitioners felt dependent and demoralized in this clinic, an experience related to differences in culture, social class, and a minority social status. Unfortunately, practitioners in these clinics are left alone to sort out this experience. Certainly no health science education program prepares health care professionals to work with the social, economic, and political intensities associated with the position of primary therapist in a rural mental health care delivery program like this one. The therapists, upon employment, were not prepared to work with the poor. They were not aware of the political nature of the rural mental health programs nor of their problem-centered history in central Appalachia. They did not anticipate the financial insecurities associated with social and health service programs in Appalachia, nor did they expect to work primarily to maintain their employment system rather than to provide mental health care.

Therapists used cultural explanations as a frustrated response to their inability to adequately fulfill the therapist role. These explanations, drawn somewhat from the earlier Appalachian community studies literature and somewhat from their own experiences and observations, were never absolute. Nevertheless, "It's their culture; people are different down here," was a ready comment when faced with the expectation of effectively and efficiently treating an impossible case load of poor and lower working-class, emotionally disturbed, rural and industrialized Appalachian people.

Ironically, the primary therapists possessed the very sensibilities needed to enhance the therapeutic dimension of their role and subsequently to make their employment more tolerable. They attempted to work within an Appalachian sociocultural framework and the sense of difference between themselves and their clients actually was a healthy one. These sensibilities needed only to be refocused toward a more problem-solving approach to clinic practice and care. The therapists made a common mistake of using the concept of culture as a synonym for behavior, a usage with limited explanatory power. Still, it is important to retain an appreciation for culture in the clinic, where it is best applied as a conceptual vehicle through which practitioners may understand the meaning patients give to their daily experiences, including the experience of illness. This understanding, in turn, should be used directly within the patient-practitioner encounter as a tool for information exchange and treatment negotiations, rather than to label patients' behavior and ultimately impair the therapeutic encounter. Therapy depends almost wholly on the abilities of the mental health practitioner and patients to mutually exchange and understand personal experiences. Therefore, comprehending cultural meaning as it infuses personal meaning is necessary to the practice of mental health care. For example, if social inequality, powerlessness, dependency, and exploitation pervade the lives of the Appalachian poor, how do these conditions affect the individual's developing sense of self, and how does an unempowered view of one's self contribute to mental illness among the region's people? There is no shortage of literature on social and political assymmetry in the Appalachian social system but no literature exists that translates the salient issue of inequality into clinical practice.

The perception of Appalachianness of the clinic encounter is most helpful when related to the difficult political and economic characteristics of employment within a rural Appalachian community mental health system. Helping therapists to objectify these real characteristics and to recognize how they impede the therapeutic objectives renews empowerment and efficacy in therapeutic encounters. Clearly, the Appalachian literature could help therapists understand the political nature of the CMHS and thus to take a less personally demoralized, more critically analytic approach to the clinic's administrative needs. What would happen to therapists' attitudes, for example, if they began to relate their own employment insecurity to that of the Appalachian miners?

Finally, the therapists' sense of difference may easily be refocused to the stark realities of disparity in social class in Appalachia, and it is useful to think of the services offered in local clinics as another addition to a long list of inequalities and inadequacies in the social options available to the Appalachian poor and lower working class. Interestingly, the nonlocal health care professionals who work at the mental health clinic have conflicts with the clients very similar to those of local professionals, suggesting that the perceived difference between therapists and patients is a class difference viewed as a cultural difference. Mental health services are an incomplete answer to the full needs of those in poverty, though to be sure clients bring the totality of their needs to therapy. Would it not be helpful if therapists were able to sort among the social complexities, only one of which is social class, that inform the varying expectations placed upon the therapeutic encounter by both patients and practitioners?

These examples bring us to a final point: Appalachian studies could be made relevant to health care professionals by regional scholars who are willing to apply their critical and academic expertise to the resolution of problems in Appalachian-based health service settings.

A PROFESSIONALLY RELEVANT LITERATURE

The majority of the literature published about Appalachia during the 1960s and 1970s was written by professionals motivated by, and in fact as a reflection of, their frustration and failed expectations. Although acknowledging the ethnographic errors and prejudices in this literature, many regional professionals today continue to read and refer to this era of Appalachian studies, admittedly identifying with the implicit sense of frustration in the authors' presentation. Unlike many of the area's academics and activists, regional professionals consequently are often unwilling to dismiss this literature as wholly erroneous.

Rather than acquiescing in their sense of frustration or criticizing the literature for an honest reaction to the difficulties associated with working in social and health service programs, I would like to see an expansion of the Appalachian studies literature to identify the sources of conflict between and the maladaptive responses of clients and professionals and to examine methods of alleviating worker frustration in the region. While the important work of advocating broadly scaled socioeconomic changes for the region in the future continues, attention must be directed to the ongoing encounters that result in demoralization and dependency in Appalachia.

Especially needed is research focusing on the effectiveness and quality of daily patient-practitioner encounters in clinical settings. These encounters are the specific situations in which the exchange of ideas and attitudes between the professional and the client occurs. Taken collectively, they have the potential of being self-enhancing or self-diminishing. For the mental health client, these encounters are repetitive and their effect accumulative. They are, therefore, powerful settings shaping self-understanding for both client and professional. These daily, repetitive, accumulative encounters must be affected by and infused with more accurate and adequate sensibilities about Appalachian people.

In the clinical setting, the patient-practitioner encounter requires a complex understanding of the Appalachian social and political context in which a health care delivery system operates (see Couto 1975, 1983; Kenny 1971), of the organizational culture and structure of the particular clinic (Jelinek, Smircich, and Hirsch 1983), and of the beliefs and behaviors the individual patient and practitioner each bring to the encounter, as well as the sources from which these beliefs and behaviors spring (Batteau and Obermiller 1983; Bledstein 1978). These complex understandings must be synthesized into a professionally relevant and reflective literature.

A professionally relevant literature calls for current research in applied settings, the analysis of which will benefit from and be informed by many humanistic perspectives. Most instructive to mental health practitioners, for example, would be a continuing series of published psychiatric case histories, comprehensively and sensitively analyzed, and published in a learning-unit presentation accessible to practitioners in local clinics and regional hospitals. Obtaining case histories to continually renew such a published series assumes, indeed requires, ongoing applied research relevant clinically and to the Appalachian community. Similarly, clinical case studies of problems and issues frequently surfacing in patient-practitioner encounters, especially those relevant to practice in Appalachia, would be instructive. Finally, a literature written for continuing professional development in Appalachia would be equally beneficial. Although professional organizations usually provide opportunities to remain viable within specific disciplines, there are no such opportunities to help professionals mature specifically as seasoned workers dealing with Appalachian people.

The achievement of professional development in Appalachia also requires a literature that is professionally reflective. A literature helping working professionals to think about their work in ways other than the routine meeting of a daily schedule is especially important in the demanding social and health service settings. This literature should help service providers ask questions of themselves as integral contributors both to the character of their work setting and to the quality of the experience clients receive. Working in Appalachia is never an arbitrary experience. Neither local nor nonlocal mental health practitioners conveyed an arbitrary attitude toward their employment relationship with the CMHC. Some were inextricably bound by emotions and convictions relating to a conscious choice to work in a locale that was also their native home. Others came to the clinic explicitly to make a contribution to a region with severe and compounded social problems. All of them took the Appalachian setting of their professional work seriously and attempted to practice with sociocultural sensitivity, a desirable and workable quality differentiating them from the narrowly biomedical, socioculturally insensitive practitioners characteristic of much of American health care delivery (Kleinman et al. 1978). These are the health professionals who will benefit from renewed efforts within Appalachian studies to more evenly inform professionals of the current critical perspectives on the Appalachian experience.

Medical practitioners are always confronted by patients' perspectives about their illness. They may find these notions quite ordinary, curiously different, really odd, seemingly crazy or, more regrettably, doctors may not hear patients' views at all, only as some extra noise in the office-bedside discourse.

But having heard those views of patients, inquisitive professionals (whether practitioners, teachers, or students) may look further. Not only do they gossip among themselves about what they know from the unwritten lore of medical practice (which is full of unsystematic field observations out of office, home and hospital visits), but they also search for books which might explain the roots of those curious notions of patients. Why does the patient think or believe that way? Moreover, what shall we do about it? [Stoeckle 1985, p. 93]

Mental health practitioners are in need of clinically relevant educational materials whose contents provide understanding beyond the biomedical perspectives conventionally applied in practice (Chrisman and Maretzki 1982; Eisenberg and Kleinman 1980). In addition, they discover by experience the need for special sensibilities when working in Appalachia. These are the same sensibilities Appalachian scholars and activists consider commonplace as they work among Appalachian people. To practitioners, however, these sensibilities are not commonplace.

To make them commonplace, it is necessary to redirect renewed efforts in Appalachian studies toward the many professionals genuinely concerned about Appalachian people and the Appalachian region, who are employed in service settings dealing with the social and health problems that continue to permeate the quality of life in Appalachia.

NOTES

This paper is based on research completed during the course of a field internship in Appalachia, sponsored by The Appalachian Internship Program, Lyndhurst Foundation, and the Appalachian Center, University of Kentucky. All place names and personal names are pseudonyms to assure anonymity.

REFERENCES

Ball, R.A. 1968. A poverty case: The analgesic subculture of the Southern Appalachians. *American Sociological Review* 33:885-95.

Batteau, A., with P. Obermiller. 1983. Introduction: The transformation of dependency. In *Appalachia and America: Autonomy and regional dependence*, ed. A. Batteau, 1-13. Lexington: University Press of Kentucky.

Bledstein, B. 1978. *The culture of professionalism*. New York: Norton.

Chrisman, N.J., and T.W. Maretzki, eds. 1982. *Clinically applied anthropology*. Dordrecht: D. Reidel.

Couto, R.A. 1975. *Poverty politics and health care: An Appalachian experience*. New York: Praeger.

Couto, R.A. 1983. Appalachian innovation in health care. In *Appalachia and America: Autonomy and regional dependence*, ed. A. Batteau, 168-88. Lexington: University Press of Kentucky.

Couto, R.A. 1984. Appalachia—An American tomorrow. A report to the Commission on Religion in Appalachia on trends and issues in the Appalachian region. Knoxville: Commission on Religion in Appalachia.

Eisenburg, L., and A. Kleinman, eds. 1980. *The relevance of social science for medicine*. Dordrecht: D. Reidel.

Eller, R.D. 1983. Class, conflict, and modernization in the Appalachian South. *Appalachian Journal* 10:185-86.

Finney, J.C., ed. 1970. *Culture change, mental health, and poverty*. New York: Simon & Schuster.

Fisher, S.L. 1976. Victim-blaming in Appalachia: Cultural theories and the Southern mountaineer. In *Appalachia: Social context past and present*, eds. B. Ergood and B.E. Kuhre, 139-48. Dubuque: Kendall/Hunt.

Fisher, S.L., J.W. Williamson, and J. Lewis, guest eds. 1977. A guide to Appalachian studies. *Appalachian Journal* 5.

Goshen, C.E. 1970. Characterological deterrants to economic progress in people of Appalachia. *Southern Medical Journal* 63:1053-58.

Helman, C. 1984. *Culture, health, and illness*. London: John Wright & Sons.

Jelinek, M., L. Smircich, and P. Hirsch, eds. 1983. Introduction: A code of many colors. *Administrative Science Quarterly* 28:331-38.

Kenny, M. 1971. Mountain health care: Politics, power and profits. *Mountain Life & Work* 47:14-17.

Kleinman, A. 1980. *Patients and healers in the context of culture*. Berkeley: University of California Press.

Kleinman, A., L. Eisenberg, and B. Good. 1978. Culture, illness, and care. *Annals of Internal Medicine* 88:251-58.

Klotter, J.C. 1980. The black South and white Appalachia. *Journal of American History* 66:832-49.

Lewis, G. 1980. Cultural influences on illness behavior: A medical anthropological approach. In *The relevance of social science for medicine*, eds. L. Eisenburg and A. Kleinman, 156-57. Dordrecht: D. Reidel.

Lewis, H. 1970. Fatalism or the coal industry? *Mountain Life & Work* 46:4-15.

Lewis, H., S. Kobak, and L. Johnson. 1973. Family, religion, and colonialism in central Appalachia or bury my rifle at Big Stone Gap. In *Growing up country*, ed. J. Axelrod. Clintwood, Va.: Council of the Southern Mountains.

Lewis, H.M., L. Johnson, and D. Askins, eds. 1978. *Colonialism in modern America: The Appalachian case*. Boone, N.C.: The Appalachian Consortium Press.

McGowan, T.A., guest ed. 1982. Assessing Appalachian studies. *Appalachian Journal* 9.

Plaut, T. 1983. Conflict, confrontation, and social change in the regional setting. In *Appalachia and America: Autonomy and regional dependence*, ed. A. Batteau, 267-84. Lexington: University Press of Kentucky.

Prucha, F.P. 1970. *American Indian policy in the formative years*. Lincoln: University of Nebraska Press.

Rilke, R.M. 1985. *The notebooks of Malte Laurids Brigge*. New York: Vintage Books.

Rubinstein, R.A. 1986. The interdisciplinary background of community psychology: The early roots of an ecological perspective. American Psychological Association, Division of Community Psychology, *Newsletter* 18:10-14.

Sovine, M.L. 1986. Traditionalism, antimissionism, and the Primitive Baptist religion: A preliminary analysis. In *Reshaping the image of Appalachia*, ed. L. Jones. Berea, Ky.: Berea College Appalachian Center.

Stoeckle, J.D. 1985. Review. *Culture, Medicine and Psychiatry* 9:93.

Thompson, R.H., and M.L. Wylie. 1983-1984. The professional-managerial class in Eastern Kentucky: A preliminary interpretation. *Appalachian Journal* 11:105-21.

West, D. 1972. Romantic Appalachia. In *Appalachia in the sixties*, eds. D.S. Walls and J. Stephenson, 210-16. Lexington: University Press of Kentucky.

Yahraes, H. 1971. A community mental health center in Appalachia. In *Mental health program reports-5*, ed. J. Segal, 90-138. Bethesda, Md.: National Institute of Mental Health.

Yahraes, H. 1973. *The mental health of rural America*. Bethesda, Md.: Program Analysis and Reports Branch, Office of Program Planning and Evaluation, Alcohol, Drug Abuse, and Mental Health Administration.

Conclusion

SUSAN EMLEY KEEFE

This volume covers a wide range of topics and findings concerning the mental health of people in Appalachia. As such, it is not easy to summarize the material covered. In fact, it might be more useful to consider the collection as it bears on the question: How can the people of Appalachia be better served by mental health practitioners and services? The contributors to this volume offer a host of suggestions based on their work in the region. It is significant that despite the disciplinary differences among the authors, there is little disagreement in the kinds of suggestions they make. Least controversial, perhaps, would be the call for more research, especially research that contributes to the refinement of the concept of Appalachian culture as it relates to mental health issues.

Specific recommendations for the improvement of mental health services in the mountains, offered by the authors in this collection, are summarized below, grouped into four topical areas: (1) the accessibility of mental health services, (2) training programs, (3) qualities of therapists, and (4) therapeutic procedures. Not all of these recommendations would meet with approval from all of the authors; some may strike the reader as inappropriate. They are offered here in the spirit of enthusiastically working toward a new approach to mental health care in the mountains. New research findings are expected to bring refinement over time.

First of all, the awareness and accessibility of mental health services must be increased in the Appalachian region. The following would help accomplish this goal:

1. A well-defined planning process is needed to achieve better utilization of new and existing services in Appalachia.

2. Service planners need to become familiar with and plan services that accommodate the sociocultural characteristics of the Appalachian population to be served. Special care should be taken to plan for equitable service delivery to all segments of the population. Follow-

up evaluation of programs should be undertaken to ensure that the planning procedure has been successful.

3. Lay persons representing all significant segments of the local population should be involved in the planning process.

4. Each mental health clinic should employ a native of the mountains, preferably from the local area, as ombudsman to the local Appalachian community. The ombudsman would be responsible for increasing public awareness of the services, providing referrals to the mental health clinic, making staff members more sensitive to Appalachian cultural traits as they affect mental health services, and helping establish rapport between the clinic staff members and community members who arrive for treatment.

5. Mental health clinics should establish close working relationships with local physicians, who must become better integrated into the Appalachian mental health referral system.

6. More emphasis should be placed on establishing outreach mental health programs in Appalachia as opposed to clinic-based programs.

7. Mental health agencies should adapt to local Appalachian cultural patterns as much as possible, in order to improve rapport with staff members as well as clients. Services that are structured less hierarchically and emphasize personalism will be most successful.

Second, training programs must be established that are culturally appropriate for the Appalachian region. To do this, the following ideas are suggested:

1. Specific educational programs should be developed for lay people, such as parent education programs, which are geared to Appalachian values and culture.

2. Special clinical training programs should be established to encourage native Appalachians to become therapists and paraprofessionals.

3. Ongoing culturally relevant in-service training programs should be provided to mental health agency staff members and professional workers. Mental health professionals should be aware of the indigenous belief system concerning mental illness and the informal means used to cope with it.

4. Clinical training programs in and around the Appalachian region need to deal with the issues of cultural differences and relevant therapeutic measures for Appalachians.

5. Also required is applied research that examines cultural differ-

ences in Appalachia and incorporates the findings in developing specific therapeutic procedures that are culturally appropriate. Emphasis should be placed on dissemination of relevant techniques to mental health professionals in the region.

Third, therapists in the region must be encouraged to develop a sensitivity to Appalachian culture and a therapeutic style appropriate for interaction with Appalachian clients, the following suggestions should be considered:

1. Therapists should develop a nonjudgmental attitude toward Appalachian culture and values; tolerance of cultural differences is absolutely necessary for successful therapy when therapist and client are from different cultural backgrounds.

2. Therapists should be observant of local culture and adopt aspects that will help them to "fit in." In other words, therapists who are not Appalachians must acculturate to some extent, learning about local speech patterns, sports, and activities, such as vegetable gardening, religious beliefs and rituals, and so on.

3. Therapists will be most successful if they work with Appalachian clients on a personal and informal basis. Joining takes time but increases the effectiveness of therapy.

4. Therapists should approach Appalachian clients as their equals rather than from the perspective of highly educated authorities.

5. Therapists should attempt to understand and become comfortable with Appalachian religious beliefs, incorporating them into therapy where appropriate.

Finally, therapeutic procedures must be appropriate for the cultural and socioeconomic background of Appalachian clients and should take advantage of existing support and belief systems. The following suggestions propose ways to accomplish this:

1. Appalachian clients, most of whom are rural and of lower socioeconomic status, require therapies that are directive, action oriented, and crisis oriented.

2. Therapy with Appalachian clients should be combined with practical advice, vocational guidance, and financial counseling.

3. Family-oriented therapy will be most successful in Appalachia.

4. Therapists should take advantage of the natural support networks of the Appalachian client. For example, family reunions and vigils at sick beds offer opportunities for "natural" healing.

5. Therapy must be consistent with Appalachian cultural values and religious beliefs. Therapists should reinforce Appalachian culture and traditions as sources of strength for the client when appropriate.

6. In rural Appalachia, nonverbal, emotional, and ritualistic forms of therapy will be more successful for the most part than verbal therapies.

7. The socioeconomic and cultural background of the client must be established prior to commencement of therapy; the therapist should know whether the client has a rural or urban background and the place of residence, the client's and spouse's occupation and education, their birthplace in or out of the Appalachian region, their religious affiliation and church location. This information could be gathered during conversation rather than with a written form. It should be kept in mind that the recommendations made in this essay best apply to rural and lower- and working-class Appalachians.

IMPLICATIONS FOR FUTURE RESEARCH

The Appalachian region is undergoing extensive change. The population is becoming more urban. Large numbers of non-Appalachian mainstream Americans are moving into the area and competing for resources and services with local people. The native population is acculturating in many ways to mainstream American life. All of these processes—urbanization, culture contact and conflict, and acculturation—are associated generally with higher rates of stress for people in the midst of the ongoing change. At the same time, there is the persistence of powerlessness in the region. The lack of control over one's environment and basic services contributes to other social problems, including such things as family violence and alcoholism. It is significant, for example, that despite strongly held religious values prohibiting the use of alcohol in Appalachia, alcohol abuse is not uncommon. One important factor mediating the stress of rapid social change in Appalachia is the persistence of many aspects of traditional culture due to the ability of a large portion of the local population to support industrialization while continuing to live a rural life-style. At the same time, value conflicts are often created and intensified in such situations, causing intrapersonal and intergenerational problems.

With regard to the study of mental health in the region, an in-depth study is needed of these processes of change and their impact on the lives of Appalachian natives, the kinds of coping strategies that emerge to deal with stress, and the types of emotional problems and help-seeking patterns that develop. Particular emphasis should be given to studies of the Appalachian family and mental health. The family is a significant source of strength in Appalachia. Yet, as authors have pointed out, the family can also be a source of strain that is all the more intense when kin almost exclusively make up individuals' social support networks. In situations of intrafamilial conflict and certain overwhelming life events, kin networks may prove to be of little help. As Dunst, Trivette, and Cross (Chapter 7) point out with regard to the birth and rearing of handicapped children, Appalachian kin networks may not be all that helpful; moreover, the Appalachian parents of handicapped children appear to have trouble initiating non-kin types of help. In Cole's Chapter 12, we have a case example of the kinds of problems that can develop within the larger multi-generation group defined as family in Appalachia, especially when an "outsider" (non-Appalachian) has married in. More needs to be known about the functions of Appalachian families and the limits of their social support. In addition, studies are needed of change in family organization brought about by the processes of urbanization and acculturation. Does the extended kin network break down with these processes or simply change in form? How do urban families in Appalachia adapt to stress?

Two other aspects of cultural change seem particularly significant with regard to Appalachian mental health: gender roles and generational relations. Gender roles have traditionally been very distinct in rural Appalachia, and social change seems to affect the roles of men and women in different ways. Not only do Appalachian men and women experience different kinds of problems as a result, they also experience the same kinds of problems differently. It would be important to know the associated impact of gender on the way in which individuals present their emotional problems to therapists. Generational differences are also apparent in Appalachia as in any society experiencing rapid social change. Young people are confronted with one set of values at home and another set of values at school; often they are forced to choose between a more secure but less prestigious (in the eyes of the mainstream) traditional way of life and a new way of life that offers higher status but requires rejection of kin and heritage.

Little consideration has been given to aspects of Appalachian culture that may provide the basis for culturally relevant therapeutic measures. Family therapy certainly has much to offer Appalachians. It would also seem that mountain religion could provide structures relevant for secular therapy, especially given the recommendation for more ritualistic forms of therapy in Appalachia. The flower service in mountain churches, for example, provides a nonverbal means of resolving conflict and reinforcing social bonds. A secular version of this ritual might be successfully incorporated in therapy. Forms of Christian counseling, needless to say, might also be highly successful in Appalachia.

Finally, research is needed that will clarify the nature of the socioeconomic and cultural variation in the Appalachian population and its impact on mental health. Most of the research thus far has dealt with rural, lower-class whites. We know little about the urban middle- and working-class in Appalachia at present or in the past. What cultural traits do they share with the rural lower- and working-class? Do urban Appalachians experience mental illness differently from the rural population? Comparative studies are needed to answer such questions. Although Appalachia is predominantly populated by whites, ethnic variation exists and should be examined. Ethnic minorities in the region, including blacks, native Americans, and people of mixed blood undoubtedly share many of the cultural differences and problems of poor white Appalachians but, in addition, suffer from racial discrimination. Therapists in Appalachia need to understand the cultural diversity in the region, but they also require practical instruments that will allow them to quickly evaluate clients' cultural orientation and select proper therapeutic procedures. Research should aim at producing instruments and procedures useful in evaluation and therapy.

It is time to begin applying comparative and cross-cultural methods of study in the field of Appalachian mental health. Assumptions about similarities and differences between the people of Appalachia and mainstream American society have gone largely uninvestigated, using standard controls for differences in socioeconomic class, rural or urban residence, ethnicity, and other social demographic factors. Only with the application of comparative studies will it be possible to speak without qualification of Appalachian mental health. In this effort to understand the diversity in the region, however, we must also seek to recognize the broad cultural patterns within which diversity occurs. An approach that, in this way, takes into consideration various levels of contrast will ultimately lead to a richer understanding of and appreciation for the region and the people in the context of mental health.

Contributors

Patricia D. Beaver, Ph.D. Department of Anthropology, Appalachian State University, Boone, N.C.

Cynthia Cole, M.A., Department of Child Development and Family Relations, University of North Carolina, Greensboro, Greensboro, N.C.

Arthur Cross, Ph.D., Department of Human Development and Psychological Counseling, Appalachian State University, Boone, N.C.

Carl J. Dunst, Ph.D., Human Development Research and Training Institute, Western Carolina Center, Morganton, N.C.

Cathy Melvin Efird, Ph.D., M.P.H., Bureau of Maternal and Child Health, Department of Health and Environmental Control, Columbia, S.C.

Judith Ive Fiene, Ph.D., Department of Social Work, University of Tennessee, Knoxville, Tenn.

Rhoda H. Halperin, Ph.D., Department of Anthropology, University of Cincinnati, Cincinnati, Ohio

Richard A. Humphrey, Ph.D., Pastor, Cherokee United Methodist Church, Johnson City, Tenn.

Susan Emley Keefe, Ph.D., Department of Anthropology, Appalachian State University, Boone, N.C.

David F. Peters, Ph.D., Developmental Evaluation Center, Murphy, N.C.

Gary W. Peterson, Ph.D., Department of Child and Family Studies, University of Tennessee, Knoxville, Tenn.

Thomas Plaut, Ph.D., Department of Social and Behavioral Sciences, Mars Hill College, Mars Hill, N.C.

Marcia Slomowitz, M.D., Department of Psychiatry, University of Cincinnati, Cincinnati, Ohio

Melanie L. Sovine, Ph.D., AIDS Activity Office, Department of Health, City of Chicago, Chicago, Ill.

Carol M. Trivette, Ph.D., Human Development Research and Training Institute, Western Carolina Center, Morganton, N.C.

Eileen Van Schaik, Ph.D., Department of Behavioral Science, University of Kentucky College of Medicine, Lexington, Ky.

John White, Ph.D., Department of Psychology, Berea College, Berea, Ky.

Index